Taking Charge
of Your Health

A Guide to
Getting the Best
Health Care
as You Age

Taking
Charge of
Your Health

John R. Burton, M.D.
William J. Hall, M.D.

THE JOHNS HOPKINS UNIVERSITY PRESS
Baltimore

© 2010 The Johns Hopkins University Press
All rights reserved. Published 2010
Printed in the United States of America on acid-free paper
2 4 6 8 9 7 5 3 1

The Johns Hopkins University Press
2715 North Charles Street
Baltimore, Maryland 21218-4363
www.press.jhu.edu

Library of Congress Cataloging-in-Publication Data

Burton, John R.
Taking charge of your health : a guide to getting the best health care
as you age / John R. Burton and William J. Hall.
p. cm.
Includes index.
ISBN-13: 978-0-8018-9551-7 (hardcover : alk. paper)
ISBN-10: 0-8018-9551-0 (hardcover : alk. paper)
ISBN-13: 978-0-8018-9552-4 (pbk. : alk. paper)
ISBN-10: 0-8018-9552-9 (pbk. : alk. paper)
1. Older people—Medical care—Popular works.
I. Hall, William John, 1939– II. Title.
RA777.6.B87 2010
613'.0438—dc22   2009038871

A catalog record for this book is available from the British Library.

*Special discounts are available for bulk purchases of this book. For more
information, please contact Special Sales at 410-516-6936 or
specialsales@press.jhu.edu.*

The Johns Hopkins University Press uses environmentally friendly book
materials, including recycled text paper that is composed of at least 30 percent
post-consumer waste, whenever possible. All of our book papers are acid-free,
and our jackets and covers are printed on paper with recycled content.

To America's seniors,

who deserve high-quality, comprehensive health care,

delivered with compassion

Contents

Preface   ix

Acknowledgments   xiii

~ PART I ~

The Older Patient in Today's Health Care System

1   Aging Today   3

2   The Complexity of Medical Care for Seniors   14

~ PART II ~

The Health Care System

3   Clinical Settings and Key Programs for Seniors   23

4   How Will the Crisis in Health Care Financing
     Affect You?   49

5   Understanding Primary Care and How to
     Improve It   60

6   Your Doctor's Perspective   75

7   Getting the Most from Your Referral to
    a Specialist   86

8   Geriatrics Education for All Health
    Care Providers   99

~ PART III ~

Managing Your Health

9   How to Take Charge   109

10   How to Choose a Doctor and Make the Most of
     Your Appointment   114

11   Screening Tests for Seniors   128

12   Managing Medications   132

13   Nutrition and Exercise   143

Index   149

Preface

Ask any of us what we value most as we age, and we are likely to mention good health. Our desire to remain healthy as we age often trumps our craving for financial security, housing, longevity, and in many cases, even life itself. The growing scientific exploration of aging has identified some of the predictors of good health. Key factors include our genetic inheritance, access to the health care system, personal health practices, and a substantial element of good luck. Because at present we cannot manipulate our genetic apparatus or our luck, we are well advised to concentrate on the other two elements: access to the health care system and personal health practices.

In this book we explain the sometimes arcane health care system currently available to seniors in the United States. To use this system in a way that maximizes our health, we must understand its strengths and weaknesses. The U.S. health care system has come a long way in understanding and caring for older people, but it is far from perfect or uniform in its delivery of that care. Seniors need to be able to differentiate the roles and expertise of physicians in primary care, geriatrics, specialties, and subspecialties. We need to understand the role of a consultant physician and his or her relationship with a generalist primary care physician. We must better understand how our physicians think and practice and become skillful communicators with our health care providers. We need to know more about our prescribed medications than ever before. Realizing that this information is hard to come by, we have written this book for older Americans who seek the latest and best information on how to maintain good health.

In addition to education about the health care system, this book offers advice on personal health practices. Today Americans are bombarded by guidance on successful aging, longevity, and anti-aging practices. Some sources are authoritative and excellent; others, sadly, can be classified only as snake oil, with little or no evidence to back up sometimes preposterous claims. In the third part of this book, we present a scientifically grounded "life plan" that we not only advise for our patients but also strive to live out for ourselves.

Who are we to presume on your time in these matters? Professionally, we are two physicians who have lived in the world of highly specialized medical care, then gravitated into general medicine, primary care, and ultimately to geriatrics. We have practiced medicine for many years and are both professors at U.S. medical schools. We have had the opportunity to teach and to learn from generations of young medical students, postgraduate trainees, and other health care professionals. Out of this decades-long process, we offer our perspective on the workings of this healing profession we love so well.

In our combined 140 years of life, we have also had occasion to be recipients of medical care. We have each personally experienced what it means to be an aging patient in the modern health care system. One gains a modicum of humility in the process.

When we began our collaboration on this book, our inclination was to address our message to medical students and young physicians-in-training. After all, we have been privileged to spend most of our professional lives at two medical schools that have championed the doctor-patient relationship in teaching and role-modeling. However, we realized that the great debate about health care reform has devoted little attention to protecting the time and space for a caring physician to work in collaboration with an informed patient. Thus, while we trust our messages will resonate with our students and young physicians, we offer our thoughts first to all who are aging or who care about someone who is.

We hope you will approach this book as if the three of us were having a conversation, enjoying that most scarce commodity in modern health care: meaningful time together for the physician and patient. We offer insights gained from our many years of clinical experience so that seniors and their families may more fully understand the nuances of our complicated health care system and derive the best from it.

As for the final element of good health—luck—we have each had our share of both good and bad. Fortunately, the good has enabled us to spend our lives helping older adults attain and maintain good health to enjoy the abundant rewards of aging. We wish you the good luck and good health to confidently offer your creativity and wisdom to the world for years to come.

Acknowledgments

This book would not have been possible without the encouragement, support, and help offered by many people. First, we thank our patients, who over the years have taught us about medicine and life with all its trials, tribulations, and wonders. We cannot imagine a more rewarding professional life. Many of our colleagues have also been instrumental in helping us develop this book.

JRB:

I am indebted to my colleagues at Johns Hopkins, especially those based at the Johns Hopkins Bayview Medical Center, where I have spent my career and where Hopkins Geriatrics is based. This academic medical center has been a nurturing and stimulating environment. I have been surrounded by outstanding clinicians, teachers, and scientists, all focused on providing ideal health care to our community and beyond.

Among these colleagues, special tribute must be paid to my mentor and friend, Dr. Philip Zieve. As my departmental chair for twenty-five years, he has encouraged and guided my career at every step. He supported and nurtured my transition from specialty medicine to general internal medicine and then to geriatrics. He encouraged the development of programs to better serve seniors, including the reintroduction of house calls. His insight, integrity, dedication, vision, judgment, and compassion have guided me and many others. It has been a privilege to receive this exceptional mentorship.

For eighteen years, I have also had the great fortune to practice medicine with Jane Marks, R.N., M.S., an outstanding nurse. Jane is admired by all for her energy, commitment, dedication, compassion, empathy, altruism, and clinical skill. She has taught me a great deal and has served as a role model for all who witness her caring. She makes the practice of medicine most rewarding.

Finally, I wish to thank both Irene Simms, director of admissions at the Johns Hopkins Care Center, and Linda Bartock, R.N.C., Geriatric Nursing home care coordinator at the Johns Hopkins Home Care Group, two colleagues incredibly dedicated and committed to the highest-quality care for seniors. Both helped collect data and provided detailed insight into the complexities of long-term care and home care.

WJH:
I am indebted to the University of Rochester School of Medicine, where I have had the privilege of being associated with some of the giants of medical education, including John Romano, M.D., and George Engel, M.D., the originators of the biopsychosocial model of medical care that has guided my professional life. Rochester is also home to the legendary T. Franklin Williams, M.D., who seems to me the perfect geriatrician and is without question an inspiring human being.

~~

We both have learned the most from generations of medical students and trainees. Through their less-dim eyes, we are constantly renewed with enthusiasm and hope for the future of medical care.

Wendy Harris, our editor at the Johns Hopkins University Press, has been most helpful. Her insights and guidance have greatly enhanced this book.

Finally, we both offer boundless gratitude to our families, who have not only supported this project but also been indefatigable in nurturing and inspiring us over the years in all aspects of our careers and our lives. Our wives, Lynda and Caren, especially encouraged us and helped conceptualize this book. Their repeated reading and editing of the manuscript have markedly improved its focus and clarity. They have both made this book not only possible, not only rewarding, but also much, much better.

The Older Patient in Today's Health Care System

1

Aging Today

Some Myths about Aging

Myths about aging are everywhere. These false notions often result from bias and ignorance, and they can lead people—*including doctors*—to overlook or mismanage true age-related problems. Laypeople and health care professionals alike carry these myths in their heads. Consider the following examples:

Myth: Urinary incontinence is a natural consequence of normal aging. True, elderly people, especially women, commonly develop urinary incontinence (about 25% of women living fully independently in their own homes suffer from this problem). However, urinary incontinence is an age-*related* disease and is *not* normal or universal. A great deal of research has led to better understanding and effective treatments for this disorder. For example, for seniors living independently who struggle with urinary incontinence and who do not have cognitive (especially memory) loss, simple educational programs alone can improve the problem for 85 percent and can entirely cure many. Yet many seniors assume that urinary incontinence is just one more inescapable burden of aging. For many, the problem becomes socially isolating, yet most of us are embarrassed to raise the issue with our health care provider. Also, unfortunately, many health care providers neglect to ask patients about this problem because they mistakenly believe it is a normal part of aging or because they feel ill prepared to help a patient deal with the problem.

Advertisements often reinforce this myth. Television commercials would like you to believe that the best answer to urinary incontinence is to wear an absorptive product or garment or to take a medication. Buried in the fine print is a required statement that urinary incontinence is a health problem that warrants a visit to a physician.

The result of this myth is an epidemic of urinary incontinence in seniors, despite the availability of effective treatments, which, for the record, almost always start with education and behavioral strategies.

Myth: Older people become bitter and their personalities change for the worse. Your personality is well established in childhood and it does not change substantially in the absence of disease. However, many illnesses that disproportionately affect older individuals *can* change one's personality. Alzheimer disease, stroke, cancer, thyroid problems, parathyroid problems, delirium, and vitamin B12 deficiency are all examples of illnesses that affect personality. *Never assume that a sustained recent personality change is due to age alone.* Missing the underlying cause of personality change allows disease to progress and can lead to disability and even death. On identifying a recent personality change in yourself or a family member, you should consult a health care provider. The health care provider and the patient (and typically the family) should discuss the personality change and its potential causes and treatments, just as they would if a lump in the abdomen were identified.

Myth: An elderly person can't exercise. In the absence of disease that might limit physical activity (for example, a devastating stroke) or disease that might be exacerbated by exercise (for example, severe coronary artery disease), all of us can exercise as we age. In fact, the wise health care provider will suggest a graded and appropriate exercise program to seniors who are not considered to be terminally ill. Evidence is now overwhelming that a regular exercise program benefits most people by improving muscle strength, relieving some arthritis pain, improving cardiovascular function, and possibly improving some mental functions. Indeed, an exercise program, even for those with severe impairment, even for those in nursing homes, can improve functional ability. Some seniors can and do develop their exercise to a competitive level. Some even compete in athletic events, including running marathons, even though as a person ages he or she can expect to run at a slower pace.

We urge all health care providers to talk with their older patients about the benefits of regular exercise, even modest programs. While it is true that some seniors ignore such advice, an exercise program is less likely to be initiated if not directly discussed during an office visit. Patients should be leery of a health care provider who suggests that the patient is "too old" to participate in an exercise program or who fails to discuss some form of exercise in the overall plan of care.

Myth: An older person can't experience satisfying sexual relationships. A great deal of research shows that while sexual interest and ability do wane with age, neither disappears. Older persons of all ages can and do enjoy sexual intimacies. However, many age-related diseases and medications used to treat these problems diminish sexual interest and performance. The effective clinician will ask a patient periodically if he or she is experiencing any sexual difficulties and, if so, will offer suggestions for further evaluation or treatment, sometimes including referral to an expert in sexual disorders.

These days one sees advertisements encouraging older people to ask a doctor for hormones, usually by injection, with promises that this will increase libido and sexual performance. Such sexual enhancement drugs have a limited role and should be used only in highly specific situations after a diagnosis of a hormonal deficiency has been established by appropriate laboratory tests. In the absence of a specific hormonal deficiency, such drugs do *not* improve sexual interest or performance. They are also expensive and have potential side effects. Similarly, erection-enhancing drugs, while helpful to many with erectile dysfunction, are not as broadly effective as suggested in advertisements.

Myth: An older person cannot learn new things. Learning can and should be lifelong, unless a person has a major brain or sensory disease. You may find that learning new things takes longer in old age than it did in your youth, but with persistence and focus it can be done. In fact, evidence is accumulating that learning not only occurs in older people but may even help delay some of the neurodegenerative diseases of old age, such as Alzheimer disease. However, studies confirming that continuing learning delays the development of disease-related memory loss need to be completed, a process that takes years. Bottom line: it is never too late to learn new things.

Myth: An older person cannot be creative. Newspapers often publish stories about marvelous creations by seniors. Such creations are known in literature, the arts, business, science, and essentially all other fields. Health care providers and family members should encourage a senior's desire to initiate a new interest. Creative pursuits build excitement and self-worth in old age, as they do in youth, and enable people to continue making meaningful contributions to society.

Myth: An older person's anemia (or heart enlargement, etc.) is due to old age. Anemia (low red blood cell count) is never due to age alone. Age-related illness, however, may be the cause. Some forms of intestinal bleeding or certain cancers, for example, may lead to anemia. It has taken years to sort out this distinction. Indeed, textbooks used in medical schools in the 1960s described an "anemia of old age." Such information was based on the results of cross-sectional studies (those that evaluate different subjects in various age brackets) that used samples of blood to check for anemia in young, middle-aged, and old individuals. Such cross-sectional studies confound the results because of the clustering of disease among older participants. More useful are longitudinal studies that follow the same carefully screened group of individuals over many years. Studying these individuals by history, examination, and testing, scientists can eliminate known diseases and determine which changes occur because of age and not because of disease. Deterioration in certain physiological functions or blood constituents can be attributed to aging only after disease has been ruled out as a cause. In the case of anemia (and in some other conditions previously attributed simply to age), longitudinal studies have taught us that all cases in older people are caused by underlying disease. Accordingly, you should challenge any health care provider who glibly attributes a new symptom or finding to age alone.

Certainly, some physiological changes, such as a decrease in nerve conduction time, maximum breathing capacity, or night vision, may occur with age, and these changes do not reflect disease. Physiological deteriorations that *are* a part of normal aging can be measured. They in themselves do not cause disease, but they do make a senior much more vulnerable to the effects of an accident, illness, surgery, diagnostic procedure, or drug and are the reason why seniors may experience one problem after another with an illness or hospitalization.

As you age, you should expect from any health care provider some recognition of age-related physiological change and the impact of such changes on your vulnerability, but disease is not attributable to advancing age alone. A good source of information on the expected normal physiological changes of aging is the National Institute on Aging (www.NIHSeniorHealth.gov).

How Do You Know When You're Old?

One of the most common questions we are asked following various public speaking events, irrespective of the topic, is: "Do you know where I can find a good geriatrician to take over my medical care?" Our standard reply is, "Why do you think you need a geriatrician?" Explanations vary but often reflect a misinterpretation of aging and of what geriatric care is all about. Invariably, these inquiries are motivated by some event in an individual's life that served as a wake-up call or reminder of her or his many years on earth.

Of course, there is no discrete threshold to old age. However, some common blunt reminders seem to signify or even scream *old!* One of the most common is the realization that others see us as old. Sometimes these reminders are impersonal, such as the AARP letter that arrives unsolicited on almost every American's fiftieth birthday. It might be the first few times a cashier asks if we qualify for a senior discount or when the discount is automatically deducted from the bill—no inquiry necessary! For others, a serious illness, such as cancer, or increasing difficulty with an established chronic illness, like heart disease, seems to suggest "old."

From the standpoint of geriatrics, the term *aging* is preferred over *old*. The aging process is part of the progression of human life, highly variable among individuals and even within the organs of the same body ("I have the lungs of a 20-year-old on 80-year-old-knees").

While it is true that a chronic disease may cause us more physical problems as we age and that cancers are more common in older adults, these disease states are not inevitable. Other changes in bodily functions *are* inevitable, though they vary from one individual to another. Such physiological deteriorations, which on average begin subtly at about age 30, do not in themselves cause disease. They do, however, predispose us to complications from an acute illness, an invasive diagnostic procedure, surgery, or another type of medical event. Gradual changes in keenness of sight or hearing, wrinkles and sags, some limitation of physical performance, and minor memory difficulties are an inevitable consequence of normal aging that all of us over age 70 would acknowledge. Persistent pain, excessive weight gain or loss, urinary incontinence, marked increases in blood pressure, or memory problems interfering with daily life are not a part of normal aging.

The field of geriatric medicine has enhanced our understanding of aging and improved the care of older adults by emphasizing how we function in daily life. Think of all the tasks you had to accomplish before picking up and reading this book. You awoke, became oriented to another day, and were probably able to get out of bed, stand, walk to the bathroom, void, wash, and groom yourself. Most of you had a reasonable appetite for breakfast. Depending on your circumstance, you may have had responsibilities for answering mail, paying bills, or driving to appointments or to the grocery store or mall. In short, despite minor complaints, you were able to function. We all observe the lessening of functional abilities resulting from inevitable physiological change and/or from age-related disease. For some of us who live long enough, this lessening may reach the point of functional limitations or frailty. However, for geriatricians, the bottom line is always how well you function in the context of any chronic diseases that you may have or physiological losses that you may have developed.

What Is Successful Aging?

Popular culture tends to reinforce many of the myths about aging. Watch a rerun episode of the sit-com *Everybody Loves Raymond* and you'll see what a battering older adults take in the entertainment media, especially television. In one episode, the dysfunctional Barone family is startled when a car crashes into their living room, driven by none other than Raymond's father, Frank. Fortunately, no one is hurt. The crash is attributed to Frank's poor vision and lack of judgment. Marie, his wife of many decades, helps play out the television version of older marital life as a hateful coexistence, caustically reveling in her husband's forgetfulness when it is discovered that he has failed to renew their auto insurance. Adding insult to injury, Frank asks his son Raymond to falsify the insurance claim to avoid liability. In the sit-com world, this is supposed to be funny—a string of tired stereotypes that cast older adults as physically fragile, cognitively impaired, socially bankrupt, difficult to deal with, and venal.

In welcome contrast, the term "successful aging" is frequently turning up in newspapers, magazines, and books. For example, the June 20, 2005, edition of the *Wall Street Journal* included an entire section entitled "The Secrets of Successful Aging." Out of curiosity, we entered the term "successful aging" into an Internet search engine and immediately found nearly five million citations!

About a decade ago, geriatrician John W. Rowe, M.D., and social psychologist Robert L. Kahn, Ph.D., published a landmark book entitled *Successful Aging,* which described the results of a nationwide study of older adults. This book presented conclusions from a comprehensive study aimed at characterizing the positive features of aging. The authors defined successful aging as the ability to maintain three key characteristics:

1. Low risk of disease and disease-related disability
2. High mental and physical function
3. Active engagement with life

Each characteristic is important, and the three are somewhat hierarchical. Good health and less disability make it easier to maintain high physical and cognitive function, which in turn facilitate engagement with life. However, Rowe and Kahn emphasized that the combination of these three components in the same person most fully encompasses "successful aging." We would add a major component of good luck to the definition. Indeed, luck affects the absence or presence of many diseases, such as Parkinson disease or rheumatoid arthritis. The major contribution of Rowe and Kahn was to emphasize the factors that we *can* influence through the personal choices we make now and in the future, the ones that do not depend on luck. They helped articulate the responsibility we can each take to achieve successful aging.

One traditional place to start studying successful aging has been with those who have achieved exceptional longevity. There is a sizable medical literature dealing with the "oldest old," those individuals 100 years of age or older, the centenarians. That Methuselah-like achievement is not a social curiosity! You may be surprised to learn that the fastest-growing segment of our population is those 85 years of age or older. The United States currently has more than 55,000 centenarians, and conservative predictions suggest that there may be as many as 600,000 by the year 2050.

Studies of the factors responsible for exceptional longevity have focused on unraveling the complex genetic factors that might predict longer life. At present, identifiable genetic factors may contribute to longevity, particularly genes that protect against many of the diseases seen more commonly in older age. Intense scientific interest is centering on how some of these genes might be manipulated, even in older people. While breakthroughs are occurring, it will be many years before the full potential of gene therapy can be realized.

Another approach has been to define the environmental factors responsible for perhaps two-thirds of the variations in longevity. For decades, researchers have carried out epidemiologic studies of groups of people who have demonstrated exceptional longevity. Some of the earlier studies have been discredited due to imperfect birth records and even fabrication of ages. However, later population studies seem to validate the factors identified by Rowe and Kahn.

The National Geographic Society recently completed surveys of populations who seem to attain remarkably long life and remain relatively healthy and robust in their communities. Dan Buettner summarizes these studies in his book *The Blue Zones*. Interestingly, these communities are found in multiple areas of the world and in a variety of ethnic groups that do not necessarily share the same genetic traits. Four places have been studied: Okinawa, Japan; Sardinia, Italy; Loma Linda, California; and the

Nicoya Peninsula, in Costa Rica. While the extent and nature of medical care vary among these sites, there are strong commonalities in the characteristics of successful aging. Specifically, these populations are similar in that there is little obesity, and diets high in fiber and low in saturated fats are preferred. These populations also engage in much more physical activity than other groups. They walk more and rely less on motorized transportation. Finally, these oldest old have substantial social involvement in family and communal activities.

When older people in the United States are studied for decades, researchers find many of the same factors at play. For example, a recent report summarized a 25-year study of U.S. male physicians who were followed to age 90. In the men who survived to at least 90 years, the actions they took to prolong their lives included: avoiding smoking, maintaining recommended body weight, and exercising daily. Happily, these risk factors are all ones that individuals, even those 70 or older, have some control over.

2

The Complexity of Medical Care for Seniors

Older persons require the best care that medicine has to offer. The older one is, the more this is true, for many reasons, but three in particular. First, with age, we gradually lose physiological "reserve" in all organ systems. Second, we tend to accumulate a variety of chronic illnesses. Third, seniors are the most heterogeneous (diverse) of any age group of patients. Thus, it is very important that your doctor exercise sound judgment and carefully consider all options in any clinical situation you may encounter. Help your doctor develop a care plan that is unique to you. Your care plan can never be right out of a general medical textbook or taken directly from a published clinical guideline. Textbooks and guidelines are relatively general and can't be applied directly to a medically complex older person, and clinical judgment must be applied to every situation. Further, the physiological changes we experience over the years can strongly influence our responses to illness and/or injury and in later years can lead to unusual ("atypical") presentations of symptoms, which make diagnosis more complex.

Physiological Changes of Aging

Longitudinal studies that track individuals over the course of decades have not only debunked many of the myths about aging but have also helped clarify the normal physiological changes that can be expected with age. Perhaps the oldest study is the Baltimore Longitudinal Study of Aging (BLSA), a program of the National Institutes of Health (NIH) that has been active since the 1950s. This large and complex research project is overseen by scientists at the National Institute on Aging (NIA). A longitudinal study, in which the same subjects participate in a series of evaluations over many years, was necessary to eliminate the biases inherent in simpler cross-sectional studies. Cross-sectional studies measure and analyze differences in different-aged groups ("cohorts") of participants; they lack the power to determine whether noted differences are the result of healthy aging or the result of entirely independent factors, such as some past environmental disruption or disease outbreak. For example, medical textbooks used in the early 1960s taught that if an individual reached the age of 80 or so years, he or she would normally experience an enlarged heart, a low red blood cell count, and memory changes. Terms like *the aged heart, anemia of old age, senility, the senile brain,* and *senile personality* were used until debunked by longitudinal studies that demonstrated that such changes were the result of superimposed disease, not normal aging.

Age-related physiologic change refers to the finding that as you age, you have less physical reserve. Such reserve is needed when you experience a bodily perturbation such as a fall, a surgical procedure, an infection, a fracture, a medication, or an invasive diagnostic procedure. This reduction in physical reserve begins around age 30, but the changes are initially imperceptible and of little importance because of the redundancy of physiological functions, the way one system compensates for another. High-performance athletes are an exception; they notice such physiological change at an earlier time in their lives. For example, studies have shown that marathon runners, even in the absence of disease or injury, experience slowly increasing times after about age 30. Professional athletes frequently retire in their forties, even in the absence of disease or injury, because they have already lost their competitive edge in performance. Older athletes can certainly perform sports such as running, including marathons, but their completion times are slower than those of younger athletes.

We all experience physiological changes associated with aging. These changes vary widely among individuals and even among different functions in the same individual. Literally thousands of such physiological functions have been measured in longitudinal studies. Examples include nerve conduction time, the excretory function of the kidneys, maximum breathing capacity, and night vision.

Inevitably, longitudinal studies are both tedious and expensive. They require that the same subjects return periodically for comprehensive testing and assessment. These reviews are currently conducted about every two years in the BLSA. At these serial visits, scientists, physicians, and technicians record a health history, perform a physical examination, and conduct appropriate testing to rule out the development of disease even in study participants without symptoms. Once disease has been eliminated as the cause of a measurably decreased bodily function, researchers can conclude that an observed change is the result of normal aging.

One reason that normal aging is important for your health care provider to bear in mind is that older people respond differently than younger people to medical tests. A diagnostic procedure that requires intravenous contrast material may result in damage to your kidneys. Also, administering new medications to you when you are older is riskier, in part because of the many age-related physiological changes. Similar phenomena were discovered about the very young nearly a hundred years ago and subsequently gave rise to the development of pediatrics and neonatology. It became clear that the young were very different physiologically from individuals in middle age, and major clinical problems resulted from evaluating and treating children as if they were small adults. Similarly, older individuals are not just middle-aged individuals with wrinkled skin. The good modern health care provider will understand and be mindful of age-related physiological changes, which steadily grow in importance with the increasing age of the patient. These physiological age-related changes are one of the major reasons that older individuals develop symptoms and signs of a new illness in a blunted pattern (for example, little or no chest pain from a heart attack) that is usually atypical when compared to what is observed in a younger individual. This makes clinical practice especially challenging among the very old. A common expression in describing the symptoms of seniors is that "atypical presentation of illness is the norm, not the exception"—diseases look different in older people.

Multiple Health Problems in Older People

Many of us who are older have more than one chronic illness. In recent decades there has been clear evidence of a pandemic of chronic disease affecting the developed world's population, especially seniors. In addition, the symptoms of, and the treatments for, one chronic disease may influence the symptoms and evolution of another.

A person may have arthritis, hypertension, vision loss, impairment of hearing, and diabetes. Another person may have hypertension, respiratory disease, and cognitive impairment. Each person, even if they are the same age, must be carefully evaluated and treated individually. Your doctor must consider your unique situation in formulating a diagnostic or therapeutic plan for you, to avoid any unexpected or unwanted outcomes from diagnostic procedures or therapeutic interventions.

The Phenomenon of Heterogeneity

There are no average seniors. Seniors are the most heterogeneous (diverse) age group of patients. If a clinician has seen one 85-year-old patient, he or she can be fairly certain that the next 85-year-old patient will present entirely different issues and circumstances, even if suffering with the same illness. There are risks to "lumping" patients by age for clinical purposes.

The phenomenon of heterogeneity leads to great difficulty in applying practice standards to those of us who are old. We routinely see the phrase "quality of care" in the headlines of newspapers and magazines. Measurement of the quality of outcomes is touted for clinicians and health care institutions, especially hospitals and nursing homes. In general, this is a good idea, but with geriatric medicine, it is not easy or obvious. While measures of quality are critically important, they are often difficult to establish for a heterogeneous population such as those of advanced age.

Consider the example of measuring hemoglobin A1C, which provides a marker of a patient's glucose control over about a three-month interval. Guidelines suggest that a level below 7 percent is an appropriate target for a person with type 2 diabetes (the form of the disease most commonly seen in seniors). Lowering the blood sugar over time to achieve a corresponding hemoglobin A1C level of less than 7 percent often requires the addition of insulin and/or oral blood sugar lowering agents, if diet and exercise are not effective. Yet relying on these agents to lower a person's blood sugar introduces the risk of *hypo*glycemia (blood sugar that is too low). Such a risk is greatly increased for an individual who has other associated problems like dementia or loss of kidney function. Hypoglycemia can be dangerous, especially if it is recurrent and/or prolonged. Also, because of variable physiological changes and chronic illnesses in an older individual, the symptoms of low blood sugar may be far less obvious than in a younger person. This is but one example of the challenges posed by the phenomenon of heterogeneity.

These three phenomena—age-related physiological change, multiple chronic illnesses in an individual, and population heterogeneity—all require that the primary care you receive as an older adult be thoughtful, unique, and carefully planned. Sound clinical judgment is universally important in medicine but is paramount in caring for seniors.

The Health Care System

3

Clinical Settings and Key Programs for Seniors

The care of those of us who have developed chronic disease or disability requires a broad variety of clinical care sites. Our health care system has become increasingly complex, and the broad range of sites offering care to seniors now requires a more sophisticated consumer. Older patients need to understand the scope and the limitations of services available at any prospective site. With a strong understanding of the various types of clinical care settings, you will be better equipped to effectively evaluate your choices.

You might be surprised to learn that many practicing physicians need the same education about the health care system. In many medical schools, there is no required course about the health care system itself. This means that you or your family must take on an even greater responsibility in evaluating one clinical setting versus another. What are the differences between nursing homes, assisted living facilities, and day care centers for seniors? What if you need extended institutional care after a hospital stay for an acute illness? This chapter is intended to help you understand and navigate the often confusing range of available options.

The Outpatient Site

The vast majority of U.S. health care is delivered in outpatient settings, either in freestanding medical offices or hospital-based clinics. In either case, the primary care provider's office should serve as the keystone of the health care system. It should be where patients initiate care and seek medical advice. Offices vary dramatically in size and some are better equipped than others to take on the important job of coordinating patient care. For older people with multiple chronic diseases or disabilities, finding the right outpatient site is critical. It is worth finding out how informed the primary practice staff is regarding services available to seniors in the community. How interested is the provider in helping patients and families sort out complex issues that require communicating with specialists? Is the provider able to offer informed referrals? One way to get a better sense of a provider's interest and knowledge is to ask a question like, "What advice can you give me regarding a local continuing care retirement community (or day care center or nursing home)?" If the physician provides no advice, then you can ask where to go to find information. The responses will give you a sense of the doctor's interest in, and knowledge about, the local care options.

Some primary care offices have only one physician and a receptionist; most, however, have several physicians and a large staff, including a technician to assist with laboratory work and procedures; a nurse (or several nurses); and often nurse practitioners or physician assistants (sometimes referred to as "physician extenders") who are trained and credentialed to evaluate and treat patients. In many states, nurse practitioners and physician assistants are permitted to prescribe certain drugs. Larger practices and hospital clinics may also have a social worker available to help patients and their families. You should be aware of the various people working in your primary care physician's office so that you know where to turn for advice. Because of the shortage of primary care physicians, it is well worth the effort to become established with a primary care provider in your area and hold on to this relationship as long as possible.

The Hospital or Medical Center

While most medical care is delivered in outpatient settings, it is the hospital, or medical center, that receives the most attention. Hospitals are the largest financial component of health care and are heavily used by all age groups. However, national data show that older people as a group, who make up about 15 percent of the population, account for nearly 40 percent of hospital admissions. Hospital size varies widely, from the mammoth and complex academic medical center to the small, rural community hospital. The resources available at these institutions also vary, usually based on the institution's size. Some medical centers have tight and formal relations with other components of the system, such as nursing homes or day care centers, but most do not, again leaving you or your family to navigate the potentially precarious transfer of your care from the hospital or medical center to another clinical site.

Hospitalists and Hospitalist Teams

Hospitalists are doctors who have a practice focused solely on the care of a patient during a hospitalization. More often than not, if you are admitted to a hospital, even by your own physician, you will be cared for during your stay by a hospitalist team. This team usually consists of a doctor working with one or several nurse practitioners or physician assistants. Most likely, you will not be assigned the same hospitalist physician from shift to shift and day to day, which may make it more difficult for you or your family to receive consistent information and advice.

In your favor, care provided by a hospitalist is more likely to be up-to-date and based on published evidence. This is ideal. Also, hospitalists are slightly more efficient in scheduling diagnostic and therapeutic procedures than generalists who come to the hospital only before or after seeing patients all day in an outpatient or office setting. In recent years, hospitalist work has become very attractive for young doctors and has pulled physicians away from office-based primary care. Most hospitalists are recent graduates of training programs.

Because the hospitalist works *at* the hospital, your access to him or her is generally easy. Evidence is accumulating that some aspects of hospital care may be better when provided by a hospitalist as opposed to a general physician. For example, as published in the *New England Journal of Medicine* (December 20, 2007), Dr. Peter Lindenauer and colleagues found that the average length of stay for seniors admitted to an acute hospital with certain common conditions was slightly shorter when care was directed by a hospitalist. Importantly, these shorter hospital stays were not followed by an increase in deaths or readmissions to the hospital within two weeks of discharge.

From the patient's perspective, however, having hospital care provided by a hospitalist as opposed to one's own, familiar primary care physician introduces complications. The transition to a different care setting after discharge from the hospital may be more fragmented, and details can be lost in transition. The hospitalist won't know you and your family as well as your own doctor does and may not consider details about you that may be important in your care. Further, hospitalists tend to work in shifts, so you may encounter two or more hospitalists during even a short inpatient stay. Therefore, you and your family will need to understand exactly who is guiding your care while in the hospital and what information is being relayed to your own doctor or, for example, to a nursing home, if transfer to one is necessary. You will need to understand how the hospitalist acquires background information about your health from your primary care provider and how information about your care in the hospital will be shared with the primary care physician upon discharge.

All too often, a hospitalization is bewildering, and people who are ill are not at their best. This is especially true for seniors. This bewilderment is magnified when a variety of new physicians, nurse practitioners, and/or physician assistants provide the care. Additionally, patients' routine medications are often changed in the hospital. Sometimes this is done for reasons of convenience or because a particular drug is not available in the hospital pharmacy, sometimes for sound medical reasons, and occasionally because of physician preference. Such changes in medications can lead to problems during transition out of the hospital unless these new medication orders are clearly communicated from the inpatient team of providers to the outpatient primary care doctor. The same holds true if you are transferred from a hospital to a nursing home or rehabilitation center. Be sure that you leave the hospital with a list of the medications you are to take.

When you are admitted to a teaching hospital, your care team is likely to be even more complicated, and it is often difficult to understand who is who on the team. Medical training consists of four years of medical school followed by anywhere from three to seven years of postgraduate "residency" training, depending on specialty. The "house staff" (postgraduate trainees) team usually includes a first-year medical school graduate, called an intern, and a more advanced medical school graduate, called a resident. The resident is usually a fourth- or fifth-year trainee if he or she is in surgical services and a second- or third-year trainee if in other medical services. During nights and weekends, it will often be a "covering" resident and/or intern who will see you if a new problem develops. There may also be a third-year or fourth-year medical student assigned to your care. This team is supervised by the "attending" physician, who might be your own physician but is more likely to be a physician assigned to the acute hospital service for a week or more. You or your family will need to work with the nurse providing your direct bedside care to identify the attending physician with whom you should talk regarding any questions about the evaluation, diagnosis, treatment, or plan for your care. Your nurse will change from shift to shift and often from day to day, but typically at the beginning of every shift your nurse will introduce her- or himself to you. Most hospitals provide business cards for the staff, trainees, and attending physicians so that it is easier for you or your family to know who is who. If you have trouble remembering names, ask for their card or write down the person's name.

While the care you receive in a teaching hospital may seem confusing, program leaders try to minimize the complexity by clarifying to you the various responsibilities of your team members. The advantage of this sort of team care is that many trained people are thinking about your health problem and discussing the best strategies to help you. Often medical school students will have more time to talk with you than residents will, and most are eager to help get your questions answered (even if they do not yet know the answers themselves). If your hospitalist asks a consulting physician to see you, you should ask the team who will consult, what that doctor is expected to do, and how his or her input will influence your care.

In sum, if you are admitted to a hospital, you and your family must take much more responsibility than in the past to assure ideal care that satisfies your wishes and is efficient. In addition to your physician's office and the acute hospital, there are several other care settings you may need.

Rehabilitation Centers

Rehabilitation centers are designed to provide intensive, short-term care focused on the restoration of physical function. This sort of care is often suggested for seniors, who commonly lose functional ability during hospitalization for illness, trauma, or surgery.

Acute Rehabilitation Centers

Acute rehabilitation centers offer patients a team of care providers, including physical therapists, occupational therapists, speech therapists, nurses, social workers, and physicians. Acute rehabilitation is intensive and requires several hours of physical activity each day, usually in the institution's gymnasium. Acute rehabilitation facilities may be located in hospitals and medical centers or they may be freestanding.

Subacute Rehabilitation Centers

Many older people who have multiple illnesses or disabilities cannot perform the vigorous rehabilitative activity required in an acute rehabilitation program as described above. Someone who has congestive heart failure, for example, or early dementia, may not be able to handle the intense expectations of an acute rehabilitation program. In this circumstance, an individual may be referred to a facility that offers subacute rehabilitation, which is less demanding.

Most subacute rehabilitation programs are part of nursing homes where a few beds are dedicated to the level of rehabilitation appropriate for an older individual who has multiple chronic health problems. While this service is important for recovery, it almost always involves a different set of care providers from those in the hospital and the outpatient office. This means that the subacute rehabilitation team may not be fully aware of your health problems and overall care needs; they may be relying exclusively on a terse discharge summary from the hospital, with information focused on the problem that led to your hospital admission. *Be sure that your primary care doctor is alerted to your transfer to the rehabilitation facility and that the facility knows who your primary care physician is.*

Nursing Homes

Admission to a nursing home is often (but incorrectly) considered the final step in care planning. Admission to a nursing home merits a great degree of coordination so that the incoming resident will receive appropriate care. The resident's concerns and goals and those of family members must be fully and carefully addressed by the nursing home physician and staff. If you are not getting information you desire, ask questions of the staff. Knowing what to expect will make the transition into a nursing home more tolerable for all.

Categories of Nursing Home Beds

There are about 16,000 nursing homes nationwide, and they vary greatly in size and resources. Nursing homes generally have two types of bed classifications: skilled and custodial. They require different levels of professional staff. Charges for these services differ accordingly. Skilled nursing must be ordered by a doctor, physician assistant, or nurse practitioner. Custodial care involves assistance with activities of daily living, such as bathing, eating, and toileting, whereas skilled care involves services such as disease monitoring, intravenous drug administration, and rehabilitation therapies.

Who Pays for Nursing Home Care?

In a nursing home, skilled services are needed only for acute health problems and are therefore covered for only a limited period of time by most insurance programs, including Medicare. Custodial care is generally not covered by insurance. Payment for custodial care is predominantly the responsibility of the individual, but those who spend down their financial assets may become eligible for Medicaid coverage for such care. Eligibility for Medicaid payment for long-term custodial care varies widely from state to state.

Some older adults have, wisely, purchased long-term care insurance for such a need. Unfortunately, most Americans have not obtained private long-term care insurance. According to the 2008 American Association for Long-Term Care Insurance (AALTCI) *Sourcebook,* eight million Americans own long-term care insurance policies, and increasing numbers of younger people are now purchasing this insurance. The cost of long-term care insurance is now high, and those with certain chronic illnesses do not qualify.

Additionally, it is usually impossible or prohibitively expensive to purchase long-term care insurance after age 65. Over time, if more middle-aged adults realize the importance of long-term care insurance and obtain it, the cost may come down.

Military veterans who meet certain criteria may have long-term custodial nursing home care services available through the Department of Veterans Affairs. Finally, such services may be covered for individuals who are residents of certain continuing care retirement communities.

Evaluating a Nursing Home

Nursing homes vary widely in size, resources, and quality of care. There is no easy way for you or your family to identify the highest-quality nursing home in your area. Speaking with the managers (including the admissions coordinators) and staff members of nursing homes, talking with other residents and their families, and reviewing the record of state inspections will help you evaluate and compare facilities. The Centers for Medicare and Medicaid Services (CMS) have a useful and popular website that provides information to help you evaluate the quality of any nursing home. This website, Nursing Home Compare (www.medicare.gov/nhcompare/), is updated every three months. It is moving to a rating system of 1 to 5 stars, in which, as with hotels, the five-star rating is the highest. Web-based information and printed materials about nursing homes are also available from state agencies on aging, usually listed in the phone book under government services.

Through CMS, the federal government has established a method of evaluating the quality of care provided by nursing homes. The evaluation criteria include: (a) delivery of care, with an assessment of required reports of staff-to-resident ratios and other quality measures (such as the number of residents given appropriate vaccines, or how many residents have pressure sores, experience weight loss, or have bladder catheters); and (b) inspections, including the evaluation of health matters (such as determining if medication or safety problems have occurred) and the adequacy of fire prevention and safety. You should use these reported data only as a guide, as there are many and often complicated reasons for a home to have deficiencies or only a mediocre rating. Nevertheless, the wise consumer will become familiar with these data and discuss them with the nursing home personnel when considering a facility.

There are other valuable ways to evaluate an individual nursing home. You can gain a sense of a nursing home by making several visits to it. During a visit, ask yourself the following questions:

- Is it clean, neat, and without odor?
- Are the staff members (nurses, nursing assistants) friendly and cheerful?
- Do the residents appear well cared for? Are they out of bed and engaged?
- Is there an activities program that looks interesting?
- Is the activities director enthusiastic and engaged?
- Are physicians present, or, if not, how often do they come to the home?
- What is the attitude of nurses and nursing assistants when they talk with residents?

Meet with the admissions coordinator and/or social worker and ask these questions:

- How are residents' new health problems handled?
- How often is the medical director at the facility, and what does she or he do?

- Is a nurse practitioner or physician assistant available full time in the facility?
- What is the turnover rate of staff members, especially nursing assistants?
- Is there a volunteer program?

The answers to all of these questions give clues to the adequacy of the institution, but deciding among facilities can still be difficult.

There are major challenges to providing high-quality care in nursing homes. Nursing homes are typically isolated from other parts of the health care system, both physically and functionally. Further, staff members' salaries are often low, especially those for graduate nursing assistants (GNAs). GNA salaries are often near the national minimum wage level, yet these are the professionals who, under the supervision of a nurse, provide the vast majority of care. The turnover of the GNA staff in most residential facilities is the highest among all health care workers, and this creates an enormous challenge in team building and setting care standards for the institution. For GNAs especially, the work is physically and emotionally demanding, as residents are often cognitively impaired or unable to be grateful or gracious and are sometimes sharply critical. Further, although training is required to obtain the designation "graduate nursing assistant," the low pay in this field makes it less than attractive to most people. Some leading institutions have developed programs to provide ongoing education and build morale for GNAs, but most homes lack robust programs of this nature.

While the United States has nearly twice as many nursing home beds as acute hospital beds, physicians and nurses receive little training in or about such facilities. Even today, the majority of recent medical and nursing graduates have never set foot in a nursing facility as a requirement of their education. Hospital social workers and private geriatric care managers can be of help, but you and your family must still seek first-hand information if you ever need to be admitted to a nursing home or other long-term care facility.

Assisted Living Facilities

There is no common definition of assisted living facilities. As a result, pinpointing their number is difficult, but it is estimated that there are nearly 40,000 nationwide. They are rapidly increasing in number and now have more total beds than nursing homes do. Assisted living facilities are available in most medium-sized and large communities. The "typical" resident of such a facility is an 85-year-old woman with several disabilities. Some continuing care retirement communities provide assisted living care for residents who had lived in independent residential units. Useful websites on assisted living facilities are www.ncal.org and www.alfa.org.

Assisted living facilities are usually freestanding; a few are part of a multifaceted care delivery system or a continuum of care offered by a single institution, such as a large medical center. Exceptions are those facilities that are a part of a continuing care retirement community or are available through the Department of Veterans Affairs. In many ways, assisted living facilities are replacing the services provided by nursing homes in past years. These institutions provide care for people who need some monitoring and assistance, such as help with medication, eating, and other essential tasks. The required number of nurses and other staff per resident is much lower in assisted living facilities than in nursing homes and rehabilitation centers. The majority of assisted living facilities are private, for-profit institutions, and many are part of a regional or national chain. Some are a part of health care programs sponsored by religious organizations.

A recent estimate of the annual average cost for a resident in an assisted living facility was about $76,000, but some high-end facilities cost much more. The costs vary greatly from one geographic region to another. There is little insurance coverage for assisted living care except for those few who have a long-term care insurance policy or who can receive care from the Department of Veterans Affairs.

In their formal training, health care professionals have virtually no exposure to assisted living facilities, and few know what resources are available. Evaluating an assisted living facility is as difficult as evaluating a nursing home, but using the strategies suggested above, you can make an informed decision.

Program of All-Inclusive Care for the Elderly

A unique variation of community-based long-term care is a national program entitled Program of All-Inclusive Care for the Elderly (PACE). PACE is a comprehensive care program that pools Medicare and Medicaid funds for seniors who are eligible for nursing home care, provides incentives to keep frail older individuals living in the community, and emphasizes preventive care and close monitoring of chronic conditions to reduce the number of hospital and nursing home admissions. Geriatricians and others working in long-term care generally view PACE programs as a model for comprehensive, coordinated care that has a seamless continuum of care venues. However, the program is small nationally, with fewer than 20,000 participants. This small number is explained in part by the need for most potential enrollees to be eligible for both Medicare and Medicaid, to live within a prescribed geographic area that enables transportation to a day care center, and to accept a limited choice of physicians. A few PACE programs have branched out and allow non-Medicaid participants to pay for these services on a fee-for-service basis. If such a program is available in your community, it is worth exploring. This is especially true if you have long-term care insurance, which most likely will pay some of the costs of this service. More information about PACE is available online at www.cms.hhs.gov/pace/.

Continuing Care Retirement Communities

There has been an enormous growth in the continuing care retirement community (CCRC) industry in recent years. Now there are close to 2000 CCRCs nationwide and they are located in every state. A CCRC is a campus-based facility that provides residential living and is coupled with health services such as primary care, assisted living, and nursing home care. Generally, these resources are available on the residential campus. Upon moving into a facility of this type, residents usually start out in independent living units. Then, if a resident develops the need for more services (such as assisted living or skilled nursing), these are immediately available on the campus. For those in independent living, a meal is typically provided each day, as well as activities of interest to seniors, such as discussion groups, interest clubs, a library, exercise facilities, and often a swimming pool. Planned trips are also usually available.

The financing of CCRCs is complicated and differs from one facility to another. Many CCRCs are not-for-profit organizations, sometimes affiliated with a religious or community organization, while others are independent. A few are for-profit organizations. Many have no formal relationship with a local hospital. Most have a relatively high entrance fee; often, but not always, this fee is returned to the resident if he or she leaves the community, or it is returned to the heirs if the resident dies while living in the community. The amount returned varies by facility and is usually prorated such that more is returned if the person is in the facility a short time and less with each year of residence. The entrance fees are typically high; most range between $200,000 and $500,000. Most residents use the money from the sale of a home to finance the entrance fee. Therefore, the popularity of CCRCs can fluctuate with the housing market. Additionally, residents pay a monthly fee. Monthly fees vary greatly and are typically adjusted annually. In some facilities, the monthly fee is *not* increased, beyond an annual across-the-board increase, if a resident requires more services. In other facilities, the monthly fee goes up for assisted living and up further for nursing home care. Anyone considering a move to a CCRC should carefully research the charges and understand which services are included and which, if any, require additional payment.

Continuing care retirement communities attract residents for a variety of reasons: they eliminate the worry and challenges of maintaining one's own home; they provide convenient social opportunities, activities, and security; and they provide immediate access to additional resources if one's health deteriorates. This wrap-around service relieves a good bit of the worry for the resident and for relatives who are concerned about their family member's safety and isolation, particularly if that parent or other relative would otherwise be alone in a private home or apartment. But CCRCs are not for everyone. They are expensive, and the price tag alone puts this resource out of reach for many middle- and lower-income people. Others dislike CCRCs because they feel that living in a retirement community is too confining and offers too narrow a population of immediate neighbors.

If you are interested in a CCRC, explore this opportunity *be-*

fore you or your partner develops a severe illness or disability. Most facilities have a screening process to assure that residents are able to function independently if they wish to enter the facility in independent living. They will reject applicants who do not meet this criterion. Therefore, getting the timing right to enter a CCRC is often difficult. In addition, most facilities have waiting lists of a year or more.

We recommend that you first decide if a CCRC is right for you and then explore the options in your community. Your primary care physician may have some knowledge of the local CCRCs, and it would be wise to discuss the topic with your doctor early in your planning. Most CCRCs request your complete medical records and often require that your physician complete an entrance form. You will want to clarify who will be providing your primary care if you ultimately decide to move into a facility of this type. You will need to visit several facilities and learn how they work, what your payments will be, and what services are available. You'll also want to get a feel for the place. Talk with residents and managers of the facility. Make repeat visits to any CCRC you are strongly considering, and be sure to go for a meal or two. Your local government office on aging can provide a list of communities in the area. Information about CCRCs can also be obtained from two reliable websites. On AARP's website, www.aarp.org, type "continuing care retirement communities" into the search box. On the American Association of Homes and Services for the Aging's website, www.aahsa.org, click on "Homes and Services Directory."

Life Care Insurance

Some areas in the United States offer seniors commercial insurance called Life Care at Home (or something similar). Other programs have developed naturally and informally in communities or apartments with a high concentration of seniors. The formal, commercial programs are similar in concept to a CCRC, the difference being that you stay in your own home. Your admission fee and monthly service fee guarantee access to institutional care such as assisted living or nursing home admission, should it become necessary. Fees for these home-based programs are far lower than those for a CCRC. Your local office on aging should have information about such a program if it is available in your community. There are great variations in these attempts to offer resources for community-based independent living, and you will have to investigate to find out which, if any, are available to you.

The Medical Day Care Facility

Most medical day care facilities are freestanding, although a few are a part of the PACE programs (described above). Medical day care centers offer a variety of services, including activities, medical monitoring, therapies, social work, transportation, and meals. Some are open every day, but most are open five or six days per week. Day care facilities cost about one-third to one-half of what nursing homes charge, and these costs typically are *not* covered by medical insurance, including Medicare. Most participants pay out of pocket or are covered by a long-term care insurance policy. However, most states do provide this service for those who qualify through the Medicaid program.

Medical day care programs are of particular value to family caregivers in need of a break from their care responsibility for a few hours one or more times per week. Choosing a day care center generally is easier than choosing a nursing home or assisted living facility, as the choice can be made on the basis of location, transportation resources, and a sense of the quality of the program. By making one or two visits and staying several hours to see the program in action, you can gain a sense of the character and effectiveness of a medical day care center. The National Adult Day Services Association offers a useful website, www.nadsa.org.

A final note concerning medical day care: the future of long-term care is moving toward "community-based care." States that are paying large sums through Medicaid to provide long-term care are increasingly advocating for community-based services for people with long-term disabilities. More information can be found by typing "communities for life" in an Internet search browser.

Home Health Care

There are two types of home health care: (1) standard Medicare-covered care provided by certified agencies (commonly referred to as "skilled, intermittent home care"), and (2) "nonskilled" or "supportive care." The differences between these two types of home care services can be confusing. Home health care agencies that are certified to provide skilled, intermittent home care have grown in size and number in recent decades. Most are freestanding, not-for-profit organizations, although some are for profit and some are a component of a health care system or medical center. These agencies operate under the direction of a physician medical director, and you will need a referral from a physician.

These agencies are able to provide many different skilled home services. Their staffs include registered nurses, certified home health aides, social workers, and restorative therapists (physical, occupational, and speech). They can provide infusion treatments, respiratory care, enteral therapy (specialized intestinal feeding), pharmacy, home medical equipment, ostomy (such as a colostomy) and wound care, and specialized educational programs in diabetes and cardiac recovery. Not all agencies provide all services.

Most skilled home care services *are* covered by insurance programs such as Medicare. To qualify for insurance payment for these services, an individual must have an acute illness or an exacerbation of a chronic illness and therefore require the services of a skilled health care professional such as a nurse, social worker, or therapist. If Medicare is the payer, the individual must be homebound unless the service being provided is infusion therapy or home medical equipment; other insurance programs may not have this "homebound" requirement.

Because the services provided involve education, the individual receiving the care must have the capacity to be taught or must have a caregiver who is able and willing to be taught about the care provided. Skilled home care is designed to restore an individual's functional ability and independence while helping him or her learn to manage the health problems. The time-limited care provided is designed to reach specific goals. The length of time for home services is determined by the admitting nurse, who develops the individual's specific treatment plan. A typical period of care is several weeks (currently averaging about nine weeks). Recertification is possible if further education is needed or if the individual's condition deteriorates.

Anyone may request skilled home care services by phoning a skilled home care agency and speaking with the intake coordinator. You can locate a certified home care agency in your area by searching online, calling your local office on aging, or looking for listings in the Yellow Pages under "Home Health Care." If you are found to be eligible for skilled home care services, the agency will contact your personal physician to approve the care and authorize the treatment plan. Your physician will then be given regular feedback about the progress of care. Home care services are highly regulated by governmental authorities with respect to the services they can provide and how they are staffed. The marked increase in the number of individuals receiving home health services through an agency in recent years parallels the marked decrease in the average length of stay in acute care hospitals.

Nonskilled, supportive home care agencies can provide personal companions and aides to help with tasks such as personal grooming, laundry, transportation, shopping, and meal preparation. Such services are paid for out of pocket unless an individual has a long-term care insurance policy that pays some portion. Such agencies can also be located in the Yellow Pages under "Home Health Care" or by consulting a community-based social worker.

Hospice and Palliative Care Services

Hospice and palliative care programs offer a wide range of interdisciplinary services for people with terminal illnesses. Most formal hospice care is provided in people's own homes. Institutionally based hospice programs may be found in hospitals, freestanding hospice facilities, nursing homes, and assisted living facilities. Hospice and palliative care services are covered by Medicare and nearly all insurance companies.

To qualify for a formal hospice program, an individual must have a terminal health condition and, in the judgment of the referring physician, be expected to live for less than six months. A physician must make the referral to hospice and authorize all the treatments provided. Estimates of life expectancy are often difficult to make accurately, and all too often referral to a hospice program is late in an illness, when the individual has only days or hours to live. At the other extreme, if an individual remains severely chronically ill but does not die within six months, another six months of hospice care is usually authorized. Contrary to what many people think, to be eligible for hospice or palliative care, a person does not have to have cancer as the terminal condition. Any chronic and progressive illness that is fatal is an acceptable basis for referral. For example, many people in the end stages of Alzheimer, heart, or lung disease may be referred for hospice care.

Home hospice services are especially valuable, because they are more extensive than those available under the usual Medicare skilled home care program. Hospice nurses have special training in caring for people who are dying. They generally visit weekly or more often, as needed, and they are available 24 hours a day. The hospice and palliative care team develops with each individual a specific plan of care designed to relieve pain and control other symptoms. The team is fundamentally focused on providing care that maximizes comfort and dignity.

Hospice programs also provide a variety of skilled professionals, including social workers, grief counselors, and clergy or religious lay persons of various faiths. In addition, most hospice programs have a large number of experienced volunteers who are able to help patients. Hospice programs often supply in-home nursing assistants when this care is required.

If a patient already has a close and effective relationship with a primary care physician and/or office-based nurse who is making house calls, the added visits from a hospice staff might confuse the patient and family. All parties involved need to understand what the relationship will be between the primary care physician and the hospice nurse and staff, including the medical director, how communication will be handled, and who will establish the priorities for care. This will help reduce potential conflict between a hospice nurse and a primary care provider, who often don't know each other.

Because hospice care is focused on providing comfort and dignity to the patient and emotional support to the patient and family, complex diagnostic services are typically *not* suggested, as the burden of these on the patient and family often outweighs any potential benefit. On the other hand, certain restorative treatments, such as physical therapy, may be provided if they can help the patient attain a greater level of comfort and dignity.

In recent years, services provided by hospice programs have been changing, and to properly evaluate a hospice, an individual and her or his family needs up-to-date information on the services provided. Such information is best obtained by having a conversation with the intake or admission coordinator of the hospice program. Information about hospice care under the Medicare program is available online by typing "Medicare hospice benefits" into an Internet search browser.

Care Managers

In recent decades, private, independent care managers (also called case managers) have become widely available. Most are independent practitioners, are usually nurses or social workers, and are available on a fee-for-service basis. Most insurance programs do not cover such services, so they must be paid for out of pocket. Care managers help families navigate the complex health care system and coordinate care. They typically do not provide direct care services but rather make recommendations and suggestions as the patient's care requirements change. Care managers are knowledgeable about local health care resources but usually are not formally affiliated with any component of the health care system. Thus, they may not be able to participate in detailed discussions about specific care activities that might occur at the time of discharge from a hospital or nursing home.

An outpatient physician working with nurses or office staff may be able to provide similar counseling as part of the ongoing primary care. Indeed, care management advice *should* be available from a primary care practice, but because Medicare does not fully reimburse physicians for providing this sort of service, it is often unavailable. Nonetheless, some of these services may be covered under Medicare when provided as part of an office visit or house call. There is interest among national organizations in fostering such services in primary care practices, especially those with many older patients. This initiative is manifested in the push to create "Medical Homes," office "homes" for medical advice and primary care which would include care management services whenever a patient's care needs change. This program is under the jurisdiction of the Centers for Medicare and Medicaid Services, which hopes to study this model in several states and, if the results are promising, to develop strategies and regulations to properly finance and expand it throughout the U.S. If the Medical Home program is broadly adopted, any primary care office designated as a Medical Home will be paid more than the basic fee-for-service Medicare fees to provide easy access and ongoing advice about health resources and care management. This sort of primary care is currently offered in some practices without additional fees and in so-called concierge practices with an additional annual charge to the patient.

Transitions of Care

Given the complexity and fragmentation of our health care system, patients are especially vulnerable at the time of a transition from one kind of care to another. As we've seen, there is tremendous variety in the range of clinical settings currently serving U.S. seniors. In part because these sites usually operate independently, problems increase around the time of transfer between facilities.

Fortunately, strategies to minimize transfer-related problems are emerging. The absence of a universal electronic medical record is currently a major obstacle to streamlining communication between health care providers. The Department of Veterans Affairs employs a national electronic medical record for its patients, and this database holds promise as a model for the private sector. Other medical centers are developing electronic medical records, but at present there is no system that links unrelated care facilities. The creation of a nationwide electronic medical record system with appropriate privacy protections has become a national priority.

We seniors are among the most vulnerable patients when it comes to transfer-related complications. Nuances of a care plan are frequently lost without strong lines of communication between provider teams. Your primary care physician can and should be helpful at times of transition between clinical sites. To be effective, the physician must have up-to-date information on the care you experienced in the institution from which you are being transferred and also be involved in providing information to the care team in the receiving institution. Unfortunately, primary care physicians today rarely provide this service, as it requires considerable time and effort and is not compensated in the Medicare fee-for-service program. Families can be especially helpful in minimizing risk during transfers by being fully informed about a patient before discharge from one facility and then communicating this information to the receiving facility. The burden of managing information transfer and supervision of care should not fall as heavily on patients and families as it does now. Repairing this weakness in our primary care system must remain a national priority.

Consider the nature of transitions between the various facilities described in this chapter. Generally, rehabilitation, subacute, or nursing home patients must be medically stable. In these facilities a patient who experiences a complication such as a high fever, difficulty breathing, or mental confusion is promptly transferred to an acute hospital. Sometimes this hospital may not be the same institution from which the patient was earlier discharged. The admission to a different hospital occurs most often in cities with several hospitals, because local emergency response systems require that an acutely ill patient be taken to the closest hospital that is able to receive ambulance cases. Sometimes, even when the original hospital is the closest, the emergency room capacity may be exceeded or there may be no bed immediately available in the intensive care unit, so that hospital will be bypassed and the ambulance diverted to another hospital. When this happens and the patient ends up in a different hospital, health care is further fragmented.

In such transitional situations, you or your family needs to call your primary care doctor at once. Let your doctor know what is happening, share as much information as you have, and ask the physician to assist with the transition of care so that critical details are directly communicated and tests are not repeated.

4

How Will the Crisis in Health Care Financing Affect You?

To understand the challenge of finding the highest-quality medical care, it is worth focusing briefly on the issue of what our health care system costs in the aggregate and how this national trend influences your personal health care. Health care financing has surely had an effect on you already, even if you are satisfied with your health care.

The current U.S. health care system is the most expensive in the world. For years, its costs have risen steadily, more rapidly than the increase in the consumer price index. Without significant reform of our system, these extremely high costs will only increase as the population ages and as more expensive diagnostic and therapeutic interventions are introduced. The growth in national health care expenditures expressed as a percentage of the gross domestic product (GDP) has risen more than threefold in the past four decades, according to the national agency that tracks expenditures (for data see CMS.HHS.gov/). In 2007,

Table 1

U.S. Health Care Expenditures as Percentage of GDP

Year	Percentage
1960	5.2
1970	7.2
1980	9.1
1990	12.3
2000	13.8
2005	15.9
2006	16.0
2007	17.0
2017	20.0 (estimate)

Table 2

U.S. Health Care Expenditures Per Capita

Year	Amount spent
2004	$6,322
2005	$7,092
2008	$7,900
2010	$8,985 (estimate)
2012	$10,110 (estimate)

total U.S. health care expenditures approached 17 percent of the GDP, a level that experts agree is unsustainable. This trend is also reflected in the steady increase in total dollars per capita spent on health in our country and in the estimates for the years ahead.

These growing expenditures might be more justifiable if there were a positive correlation between higher spending and better clinical outcomes of care. Yet there is growing evidence that the opposite is more often the case. Indeed, in the United States, greater health care spending is correlated with worse clinical outcomes.

These high costs cause most organizations—small, medium, and large—that have health insurance plans to struggle. It has become increasingly difficult for businesses to provide health insurance benefits for their employees and retirees. Employers are now looking at ways to control these costs, including cutting health benefits once planned for or promised to retirees. For the first time in U.S. history, businesses as well as consumer advocacy organizations are calling for comprehensive health reform. In 2008, nearly 50 million Americans had no health insurance, and millions more were underinsured (meaning they had health insurance that proved inadequate for their needs when they became sick or injured). These numbers have continuously risen and, without reform, are expected to keep rising.

How does this national health care crisis affect seniors, essentially all of whom have coverage in full or part through Medicare? It does so in many ways: (a) the priority for adequate payment for care of older persons competes with the need to insure all Americans; (b) without increased incentives for physicians to choose careers in primary care, competition for existing primary care providers is likely to increase; (c) crowding of emergency departments (EDs) increases as the growing number of uninsured people have no other access to medical care; (d) failure to provide preventive and primary care to younger citizens who lack insurance makes it likely that more will enter old age with chronic health problems; and (e) people who lack health insurance and access to primary preventive care often show up in emergency rooms requiring hospital admission for conditions that could have been managed earlier and at lower cost. Hospitals in many parts of the country are pushing the maximum inpatient capacity, and this makes it more difficult for an older person to be admitted without experiencing delays. If hospitals respond to this capacity problem by expanding the number of beds through new construction, this will only further increase the overall cost of health care.

When there is inadequate or no reliable access to primary care providers, people turn to emergency departments as a stopgap resource. EDs are expensive sites of health care delivery and are designed to respond to emergencies and life-and-death situations. Further, EDs are struggling to provide occasional care to uninsured people, especially in large cities. The result is that EDs are congested and have long waiting times, typically several hours. These long waits fall most heavily on older individuals whose chronic disease is out of control, because in the context of the ED, their problems appear less urgent. Additionally, the subtleties of adjusting medications and otherwise working to obtain control over an exacerbation of chronic disease is not what ED physicians have been trained to do. Many emergency room professionals seem to view older individuals as crowding the departments and preventing them from achieving their primary goal of managing true emergencies. These factors add up to make EDs highly inadequate for providing primary care services for older people who are ill. The ED is *not* intended to provide primary health care, provide ongoing care for chronic health conditions, coordinate care, or offer health maintenance services.

Medicare

The Medicare program is one of our nation's great legislative successes and an enormously important health insurance program for seniors and some others. It was not always available. Early in our training, we witnessed some aspects of senior health care before Medicare was implemented. Frankly, health care was terribly inadequate for impoverished and even lower- and middle-income older patients with catastrophic illness or chronic diseases who no longer had health insurance provided by an employer. Patients with meningitis were being sent from private hospitals to city charity hospitals because they had no insurance; many seniors were lined up in free or low-cost city or hospital clinics to have their high blood pressure treated; and many people had no primary care because they couldn't afford it and would not tolerate the insufficiencies and dehumanization frequently experienced in free clinics. These were dark times for the care of many seniors.

It is easier to understand the current strengths and weaknesses of the Medicare program by recognizing that it was a concept influenced by the social and scientific realities of post–World War II America. Life expectancy was 67 years for men and 72 years for women (compared to 78 and 82 years, respectively, today). There were relatively few effective medical and surgical interventions for people with multiple chronic illnesses. Indeed, most people didn't live into their 80s, the time of life most affected by chronic disease. Therefore, the Medicare insurance program had little need to cover the costs of prescription drugs or the costs of the time health professionals now spend in chronic disease counseling, patient and family discussions about care options, and the coordination of care provided at multiple sites. The program was primarily focused on acute or short-term health care needs. At that time, hospital care was also simpler. Sophisticated diagnostic procedures were relatively few in number, and overall health care costs were far lower. Long-term care was not thought to be affordable or necessary because relatively few people lived long enough to have severe chronic and disabling disease. Not surprisingly, the Medicare health insurance program provided financial coverage mainly for acute hospitalizations and physician fees in the hospital and the office. Almost no reimbursement was provided for preventive services, most of which had not yet been shown to be effective for adults over age 65.

In short, Medicare was designed with the assumptions that we would not live long after age 65 and that serious illnesses would require hospitalization as the major intervention. Most experts now believe that Medicare must be substantially reformed to provide the care that is needed by a growing population of older adults. Life expectancy is now significantly greater, and highly effective medications and other treatments have emerged. Complex chronic disease has become more prevalent than acute illness, and the need for institutional, long-term care at some stage of life is now probable.

When our patients are approaching the age of eligibility for Medicare, we like to make them aware of some of the key components of Medicare health insurance. First, we emphasize that, while far from perfect, Medicare is a good health insurance program for older adults. It offers considerable freedom in the selection of physicians and hospitals (at least, for those enrolled in the fee-for-service form of Medicare), and it is more accepted in the 50 states than almost any other form of health insurance. We also inform our patients that Medicare was never intended to pay for all medical expenses, and for most people who can afford it, some form of supplemental (or "Medigap") insurance is desirable. Very poor individuals may be eligible for Medicaid (the federal and state health insurance program for low-income individuals) and are able to use this program as a form of gap insurance. The income eligibility level for Medicaid varies by state and may change from year to year.

Next, we make sure that patients understand the various types of Medicare coverage. Medicare Part A pays for part of acute hospital costs and some services after discharge, such as home health care, hospice care, and relatively short-term stays in a skilled nursing facility following a hospitalization that has lasted a minimum of three days. Enrollment in Medicare Part A begins automatically with Social Security benefits, as long as you or your spouse has been employed for a total of at least 10 years or 40 quarters (these quarters need not be continuous) and is a citizen of the United States. Part A does not cover extended nursing home care except for limited, short-term care. One of the most common misconceptions among Americans is that Medicare covers the costs of long-term care; it does not.

Medicare Part B partially reimburses physician fees, some mental health care fees, and, when ordered by a health care professional, laboratory tests, imaging studies, rehabilitation services, and selected preventive services. Medicare Part B requires a separate application and has monthly fees that you must pay. Part B will reimburse your physician for visiting you in a nursing home for a periodic routine visit or for an acute illness when he or she is summoned urgently. In most states, physicians can opt out of Medicare payment systems. In these cases, they will bill the patient, who is then required to seek partial reimbursement from Medicare.

Medicare Part C refers to health care plans, such as Medicare Advantage Plans, administered through health maintenance organizations (HMOs) and preferred provider organizations (PPOs). Such organizations contract with Medicare for a monthly payment and commit to providing certain levels of health care services for patients enrolled in their program. The benefits vary from plan to plan, and it is essential for the careful consumer to do comparative shopping.

Medicare Part D covers part of the costs of prescription drugs and requires the selection of a drug plan provider. Providers vary widely from region to region and do not all cover the same medications. It can be helpful to consult a pharmacist in the selection of a plan. Part D was never intended to cover all the costs of prescription drugs, so, in addition to the monthly premium, there can be substantial out-of-pocket costs, depending on the drugs prescribed and whether they are brand name or generic. The formulas for projecting these costs can be complicated. Useful information is available through the Medicare website (www.Medicare.gov) or in print material that can be ordered from the website. Another good resource is the Medicare Rights Center, whose mission is to ensure access to affordable health care for older adults and people with disabilities through counseling, educational programs, and public policy initiatives (www.medicarerights.org).

Most adults should learn about Medicare supplemental, or Medigap, insurance. Selection among the various plans can be exceedingly involved. The best source of information on selecting a plan is provided by the Medicare Administration (www.medicare.gov). You can download a detailed explanation or order a print copy. In weighing these plans, remember that it is best to purchase a plan during what is called the open enrollment period, usually defined as the first six months after signing up for Medicare Part B. During that period, insurance companies must accept any applicant regardless of preexisting health conditions. If you wait beyond the open enrollment period, companies can (and often will) adjust coverage and rates. All Medigap policies are sold by private insurance companies. They are standardized policies that must comply with both federal and state regulations.

We encourage you to consider the Medicare preventive health benefit that was added in January 2007. Within the first six months of reaching entitlement age (usually age 65), each Medicare participant is eligible for a "Welcome to Medicare" visit to his or her primary care provider. This visit provides key preventive health services as well as the development of a preventive plan for the future and is well worth the time and small charge.

Since 1965, at the inception of the Medicare and Medicaid programs, there have been universal health insurance programs for citizens aged 65 or older, some younger individuals with disabilities, and very poor people. Medicare and Medicaid have been vitally important; these programs greatly improve the health and well-being of the populations they cover. They have eliminated the indignity that was often suffered by those seeking no-cost or low-cost health care before 1965. Studies published in the *Journal of the American Medical Association* (December 26, 2007) and the *New England Journal of Medicine* (July 12, 2007) showed that health care improves in important ways for previously uninsured individuals after they turn 65 and receive Medicare coverage.

The Need for Health Care Reform

Despite the advances brought by Medicare and Medicaid, these programs have not kept up with the times. Medicare and Medicaid programs were implemented at a time when life expectancy was in the high 60s and death typically resulted from acute illness. The health profile since the 1960s has changed dramatically. Today, those who reach the age of 65 have, on average, nearly two more decades to live. Now chronic disease, not acute illness, is the most prominent challenge facing older patients. Medicare needs to be updated and modified to more effectively serve the needs of its enrollees. Many people have advocated for such reform, yet nothing can happen without the leadership of our national government because so much of the U.S. health care system is intertwined with government-sponsored programs. Indeed, no major private sector health care initiative has had much effect on the health care of seniors in recent decades.

The difficulty with governmental leadership, according to many, is that too frequently elected officials don't act in the best interest of the public. Experts explain that politicians are unduly influenced by the tremendous lobbying efforts of industries that profit from the status quo. Interest groups that have traditionally slowed or blocked efforts at substantive, patient-centered reform include hospital groups, physician groups, insurance companies, drug companies, and medical device manufacturers. Influenced by pressure from this well-heeled collective, Congress has failed to initiate health care reform in recent decades, leaving millions of people without access to good-quality, affordable health care. In the absence of national leadership on this front, several states have taken it on themselves to pass legislation and identify funding to provide better health care for their residents. These sorts of state initiatives, while noble and forward thinking, are now put at risk by the strain of economic recession on state budgets.

As this book goes to press, vigorous federal health care reform is developing. It is imperative that constituents let their elected officials know how important it is to protect and promote primary care and to ensure that Medicare's reimbursement rates for such providers are high enough that they are not deterred from seeing Medicare patients. We encourage you to communicate with your local and state representatives and to work with the health care committees of major organizations like the AARP.

Health care reform has become a major priority for our country, for both economic and moral reasons. Sustained leadership is necessary to continue to move health care reform to fruition, and it is up to all of us to keep our leaders focused on this most urgent crisis. Perhaps more than ever before, consensus in the United

States is building to achieve the needed reform in health care. Compromise will be necessary to achieve meaningful success, and those of us with vested interests must focus on the health care of all citizens above our own special interests.

5

Understanding Primary Care and How to Improve It

Primary care providers are at the heart of coordinated health care. These providers help patients maintain good health and, when illness or injury strikes, they are the first to turn to for help. They are able to connect patients with specialist physicians and follow up on the results of those visits. Having a physician provide ongoing surveillance of this nature is of great value. Your primary care provider serves as your health advisor and should be the first health professional you consult when faced with any new symptom or problem that is not a life-threatening emergency. Increasingly, nurse practitioners and physician assistants are joining primary care medical practices as primary care providers.

Among physicians, primary care is ideally provided by generalists: general internists, family physicians, geriatricians, and, for children, pediatricians. The training, orientation, and experience of generalists are focused on providing primary care. These generalists are positioned to be the point of access to the system, to help patients deal with new symptoms or health events, and to coordinate the care for multiple chronic problems and health maintenance issues.

The generalist physician has a broad vision and approach to analyzing your symptoms and knows when it is appropriate to consult with specialists. Seniors frequently have multiple health problems compounded by losses of physiological reserve, making them one of the groups of patients most vulnerable to illness or injury. Many individuals who have a health problem that is predominantly limited to one organ system (for example, heart failure from coronary artery disease) receive all of their care, including primary care, from a specialist (in this example, a cardiologist). While this form of care is entirely satisfactory for some patients, it is not ideal for seniors because specialists, with their targeted focus, may not be sufficiently knowledgeable about your other health issues.

The ongoing relationship that you have with your primary health care provider ensures that acute and chronic health problems are dealt with promptly. In this relationship, you should receive a thorough explanation of all of your health issues so you understand your primary care provider's thinking about your health and the recommended evaluation and treatment of any problem. Your primary care provider should be able to advise you regarding health maintenance and preventive health services. Your primary physician or an associate or staff member should be available to address any health- or medication-related question or concern. Most often for older individuals, a routine scheduled visit to a primary physician includes all of these elements. For example, if you are an 85-year-old, your visit should include: a response to all your concerns, an assessment of your major health problems (such as diabetes, hypertension, vision loss, arthritis, depression), a review of your medications, an assessment of any new symptoms or changes in your functional abilities, a review of any changes in your family or living situation, and a review of appropriate preventive health strategies (such as immunization status, diet, and exercise). Some of this may be determined by the other staff and then communicated to the doctor. Ideally, a primary care provider should work in a system that has 24-hour, 7-day-a-week access, to respond to urgent health issues that might develop. This does not mean that the primary care office should be continuously open, that it should replace the emergency department of a hospital, or that it should serve as a freestanding urgent care facility. However, the primary care physician or a designated surrogate should be always available to provide direction on how to handle an urgent problem. The primary care provider is not simply the professional who helps an individual with colds and minor problems. Rather, the primary care provider's responsibility is, on a continuing basis, to evaluate your symptoms, provide ongoing care and advice for all your acute and chronic conditions, and offer guidance regarding preventive services.

Older people, especially those who are over 80, require the best of primary care, someone keeping tabs on their entire health picture. This is because of the substantial loss of physiological function that accompanies normal aging, the accumulation of multiple illnesses, and the variability typical of seniors. This combination of clinical characteristics makes the very old population the most vulnerable of any group (other than the very young) and highly subject to complications from diagnostic and therapeutic interventions. Indeed, hospitalization in and of itself puts the older patient at a much higher risk of an adverse outcome than nearly all other age groups. For this reason, older patients require the most sophisticated, accomplished, and thoughtful primary care possible. Good judgment by practitioners must be a core component of health care for seniors. A test for one problem could easily have an adverse effect due to other, age-related medical and mental problems and loss of physiological reserve. Because of these issues, the care of older people takes extra time, judgment, and broad knowledge.

A recent clinical experience illustrates the need for expert primary care for older people. An 87-year-old woman who lives alone has osteoporosis, hypertension, heart failure, mild kidney disease, arthritis in her knees, visual impairment, and fluid retention. She came to the office with abdominal pain that was new for her. A CT (computed tomography) scan of her abdomen would require her to temporarily stop drinking fluids and to receive a potentially toxic contrast agent; these requirements could lead to dehydration and/or harm to her already damaged kidney. (An abdominal CT done without restricting fluids or contrast dye is safe but typically less useful.) This patient had virtually no way to get needed help at home if she had to have a colonoscopy or upper gastrointestinal endoscopy, and hospitalization would almost certainly lead to reduction of her physical capabilities and of her independence. So her doctor had to apply judgment and discuss with her a rational plan of evaluation and management of her symptoms. It took time and care to weigh the risks and benefits of procedures and treatments.

While specialists are often a core part of a senior's health care team, their approach may be more aggressive than that of a generalist physician. The specialist may be quicker to order diagnostic tests or to prescribe treatments, while the generalist may adopt a more cautious approach, with repeated office visits and longer periods of observation, potentially saving the patient distress and damage from adverse reactions to the tests or treatments.

Team Care in Primary Care

Multidisciplinary care, or team care, involves a group of professionals in the care of a single patient. In geriatric medicine, this is the norm rather than the exception. For you, this may at first seem confusing, but it generally is superior to care from one health care provider working alone. Multidisciplinary care in geriatrics is provided in all clinical settings: office, outpatient clinic, hospital, and residential facility. Composition of the team may vary, but the group almost always includes a physician and a nurse. Often, especially in institutional care settings, others are involved as well, including nurse practitioners, physician assistants, social workers, therapists, pharmacists, psychologists, or dentists. In office practice, the typical multidisciplinary team consists of a nurse and physician(s), but increasingly a nurse practitioner or physician assistant is also present.

The value of team care is that the accessibility, wisdom, judgment, and knowledge base is greater in a team than in a single practitioner functioning alone. Each health care professional brings to a clinical issue a slightly different and valuable perspective. However, for a team to function effectively, there must be training and a clear system of communication that allows for frequent, highly efficient time in a "huddle." This communication becomes increasingly complex as the team grows. With today's ability to communicate via e-mail, text message, fax, electronic medical records, and phone, a team does not need to meet in person to be effective. In fact, the team can often meet more frequently when that meeting is "virtual" rather than face to face.

In our experience, the patient or family member typically is put in touch with the nurse when calling about a new issue. The nurse gathers the preliminary information, makes initial suggestions, and then communicates with the physician or nurse practitioner/physician assistant. For example, "Mrs. S is having new pain in her back," or "Mr. C fell two days ago." A decision is made as to how to proceed: "Let's arrange to see Mrs. S urgently and, if necessary, plan an appropriate imaging procedure while controlling her pain"; "Mr. C seems to have tripped, and it doesn't sound as though he has a serious injury. Let's treat the pain and discomfort with acetaminophen and carefully applied heat, then plan to call him every day to see if the problem resolves or worsens or if new symptoms develop that warrant immediate action on our part."

This trusting and highly functional partnership within a team markedly improves the accessibility of the team, even when some of them are out of town. It enables the team to reassure the patient from a distance. This is best exemplified by a recent experience one of us had while attending a three-day medical meeting. The physician and primary nurse partner in the practice exchanged seventeen e-mail messages, four text-paged messages, and two phone calls. We were able to avoid referring a patient to an emergency room. A trip to an emergency department is expensive, time consuming, and too often a frightening experience that most old people would like to avoid except in life-threatening or extreme situations (such as passing a kidney stone). A patient's communicating with the practice nurse does not lead to a delay in dealing with emergencies. Patients often make wise decisions about when to go directly to an emergency room (for example, with the onset of severe chest pain, symptoms of a stroke, or suspicion of a broken bone).

There are disadvantages in multidisciplinary team care as well, however, most of which relate to inadequate communication within the team. Effective communication requires collective trust and knowledge, which come only with time. For this reason, teams that have frequent turnover in membership sometimes lack the effectiveness of more stable teams.

Sometimes, members of fragmented teams may explain things differently or with different emphases, and this can lead to confusion in the minds of the patient and family. Most clinicians have developed strategies to work effectively with unfamiliar health care professionals, but it is never as effective as being part of a team that works together regularly. Medical practitioners need to be trained in team communication and relationships, but unfortunately there is little training in multidisciplinary team dynamics. You will know how well a team is functioning by the consistency of the message you receive from various team members and by their reassurance to you that they have been in touch with each other and are all familiar with the details of your personal situation.

Many patients carry with them a romantic image of the solo practitioner and worry that multidisciplinary primary care is a dilution of that ideal. They think of the iconic family doctor who had an office in his home, who knew all about the family, provided care to all, made house calls, saw patients every day and often for an hour or two in the evening, and provided care in the hospital and the nursing home. Usually the family doctor had no staff, often gave out a short-term supply of commonly used medications, and collected a few dollars in cash at the end of a visit. Such individuals may still exist, but they are the rare exception. Medicine has become far too complex for a return to such practice. The cost and complexity of billing in and of itself has all but eliminated the solo physician or nurse practitioner. Further, the diagnostic tools available today require referrals to multiple specialists and institutions, and the processing of prescriptions brings its own complexities. All of this requires administrative staff assistance. Finally, in the last fifty years of medical practice, two major phenomena have eliminated the viability of the solo practitioner: the demographic makeup of patients who are ill, and the changing nature of our illnesses. Now most visits to the doctor are made by seniors, whereas a century ago, few people lived past seventy. Sixty years ago, the average age of a patient visiting a general internist was about 45, and now it is about 70. When we started in medicine, the usual primary care practitioner managed acute illnesses for the most part. Today, chronic disease is more common. Ideal primary care no longer resembles a Norman Rockwell painting.

The challenge now is to preserve and enrich patient-centered primary care even as we incorporate modern technologies. We must hold on to what is good and important in the relationship between a patient and a provider: access, knowledge, familiarity, compassion, comprehensiveness, and judgment. It is difficult but certainly possible to find a primary care physician who combines the best of the old with the best of the new. As we've mentioned, the number of primary care providers has been falling dramatically in the United States. In the near future, the public will have to insist on increased numbers of high-quality primary care providers. Now that health care is no longer solely regulated by a free market system, we all must work with government officials and large health care organizations to insist on the best in primary care. Indeed, we must develop the strategies to attract trainees to, and sustain them in, primary care practice.

There are other disadvantages to team care, but in our experience they are of minimal importance. The cost of providing team care is a theoretical disadvantage. This typically is a problem in fee-for-service practice in the Medicare program, where payment mechanisms have been built to center on the individual provider. Therefore, the amount of revenue generated is based on the complexity of the health situation and the time the patient spends face to face with the person who bills for the service. In a managed care health insurance program (also called capitated or prepaid health insurance), such as Medicare Advantage, these restrictive payment rules do not apply, and it may be easier to use commonsense and innovative approaches to care. The added expense of having a nurse-physician partnership is worth every dollar: quality of care is typically improved; patient satisfaction is usually higher; office efficiency improves (for example, when a nurse takes elements of the medical history or explains medications, freeing up physician time for other clinical work); follow-up and communication is more efficient and timely; and the nurse can communicate with a consultant or contact a pharmacist or therapist about a specific issue while the physician is talking with the patient about other issues. Administrative staff members can and should perform some of these critical functions in office- or clinic-based primary care. A nurse, however, has a deeper understanding of the nuances of the care issues and typically is able to accomplish such tasks more effectively.

If there is a multidisciplinary team in the primary care practice you use, you should find out who its members are, how they relate to one another, and how you can expect them to relate to you. In time, most patients figure this out by experience, over the course of years. We believe that knowing about these relationships can only improve the care a patient receives, and we therefore recommend that patients ask about these issues early in a primary care relationship. Multidisciplinary team care is common today and will likely become increasingly so. The models of primary care delivery mentioned in other chapters, such as "guided care," the "Medical Home," and the Program of All-Inclusive Care for the Elderly (PACE), are all multidisciplinary care programs, and each requires that in the initial encounter, patients are familiarized with the way the team works.

Only a few medical training programs actively *teach* multidisciplinary care. As citizens and a potential patient, you can have a role in urging elected officials to support such training. One model, perhaps the best known and the largest, is the Geriatric Education Center (GEC) program of the Bureau of Health Professions, which is managed by the Health Resources and Services Administration of the U.S. government. The GEC program now consists of about fifty programs, whose collective goal is to teach geriatrics to a multidisciplinary health professional audience, particularly to professionals working in medically underserved areas. Unfortunately, this program has had its funding stopped, then restarted, only to be threatened again by government officials, including our elected representatives, who are struggling to determine funding priorities when the nation's needs are so broad and great. Such fluctuating support is destructive of a program that most believe is needed, successful, and worthy of major expansion, given the dire situation in U.S. health care. Programs such as the GEC and institutions such as the National Institutes of Health—especially the National Institute on Aging, which emphasizes research—are in great need of expanded federal funding if the health care needs of seniors are to be met ideally.

The Crisis in Availability of Primary Care

The growing shortage of primary care physicians in the United States is laying the groundwork for a crisis, if not a catastrophe, in health care. One way to quantify the primary care shortage is to note that in 2007, approximately 250 physicians entered training in geriatrics, while more than 1,000 entered programs in cardiology. The predicted result is that by 2025 our nation will need 35,000 to 44,000 more adult care generalist physicians than it has. While well-trained physicians in all specialties are needed, proportionally more primary care physicians are desperately needed. This is particularly true for seniors. If an older person is not already established with a physician, he or she is likely to have difficulty finding a generalist physician to provide ongoing primary care. This difficulty is likely to worsen substantially, because the number of trainees entering primary care disciplines has been steadily decreasing in recent years.

Money has a lot to do with this crisis in primary care. Proportionately more physicians are entering specialty (and subspecialty) disciplines, such as radiology, emergency medicine, dermatology, anesthesiology, and the subspecialties of internal medicine (cardiology, gastroenterology, pulmonary medicine, and so on). The average income of a generalist, while substantial, is much lower than that of a specialty physician. The average earnings for certain popular specialties and subspecialties are now four or more times greater than that for generalist physicians. This disparity in earnings directly parallels the interest among U.S. medical school graduates in entering these respective practice fields. Studies showing salary discrepancies for medical school faculty point out that the increase in income over recent years has been lowest for generalists, especially geriatricians. To most people, salaries for physicians seem high, and indeed, physicians are living in one of the highest income brackets. This does not change the fact that many medical students approach graduation with enormous debt from their tuition costs and do consider their future earning potential when weighing career options. The *New England Journal of Medicine* (December 18, 2008) reported that medical student indebtedness recently set a new record: 87 percent of all recent graduates have debt and, strikingly, nearly a quarter of all graduates have a debt greater than $200,000. Additional financial factors influence students' choice of practice area. The high cost of staffing and maintaining an office practice also contributes to the decline in numbers of medical graduates entering a generalist discipline. Many physicians believe they will not be able to make ends meet with the limited compensation provided under Medicare. Physicians' compensation should be more balanced across the various practice fields to make primary care more attractive.

In recent years, many generalist physicians have restricted their acceptance of Medicare participants because older patients require more time and because the reimbursement levels are relatively low. In many instances, payments are not adequate to cover the increasing costs of staffing administratively complex practices. More complexity in office practices is related to the variety of billing requirements for different insurance programs and the associated paperwork. This limiting of Medicare patients makes for long waiting times for seniors to get an appointment.

The public needs to be aware of these workforce issues if we are to find solutions. One approach to recruiting more students to primary care practice is to reinvigorate training for generalists in traditional medical schools. Another is to recognize the important role of osteopathic schools, which emphasize training of generalist physicians. (Osteopathic physicians [DOs] are more common in some states than others, reflecting historical trends in state licensure.) We should also provide incentives for the expansion of these and all other schools that focus on primary care training.

The scarcity of geriatricians has prompted many leading geriatricians to call for reclassification of geriatrics as a specialty, and many have suggested that geriatricians limit their practices largely to performing consultations. Our view is different. We believe that geriatricians can use their special skills most valuably as generalist primary care providers. We geriatricians must think about, evaluate, and guide patients comprehensively, not drop into patients' care as consultants. One's practice reflects a day-after-day consistency in philosophy, style, and manner. Our own early professional experiences as specialists and largely as consultants taught us the differences in attitude, focus, and style of interaction between specialists and generalists, and we strongly believe that geriatricians are and should remain generalists.

However, this is not to imply that geriatricians should be the exclusive primary care doctors for older people; there are not enough geriatricians for that to be possible. In addition to being primary care physicians, geriatricians should teach, do research, and develop innovations to improve the care of seniors.

Finally, geriatricians as a group are heavily involved in teaching primary care, and one cannot teach the concepts of quality primary care effectively unless one approaches medicine with a primary care perspective. In short, we should practice what we preach.

Other factors that dissuade students from choosing general medicine or geriatrics include the lack of role models, the comparatively low prestige of primary care, and the sense that the lifestyle of generalists leaves little time for family and nonprofessional activities. The solutions to this shortage will require national leadership and the influence of governmental agencies. These have been largely lacking as the nation struggles with other colossal problems. Our elected officials need to continue to be strongly engaged in advocacy for increased recruitment of generalists if we are to avoid the impending catastrophic shortage of primary care providers with sufficient training in geriatrics to meet the primary health care needs of the growing population of seniors.

Solutions to the Primary Care Problem

Other professionals, especially nurses, nurse practitioners, and physician assistants, will help meet the challenge of providing high-quality primary care to seniors. However, primary care physicians must be a part of such team care, especially for the oldest individuals. A physician working in a multidisciplinary primary care team must have the experience, focus, and training consistent with providing primary care. Most specialist physicians, while perfectly capable of working in teams with other health care professionals, do not have this primary care background or focus.

Programs have been created to make up for the lack of high-quality primary care. One increasingly popular style of practice is *concierge medicine*. In this model, the patient pays a substantial annual out-of-pocket fee to a physician to guarantee timely access to, and coordination of, care. In addition to the annual self-pay concierge fee, visits and procedures are billed to the patient's insurance program, usually Medicare, as in a non-concierge practice. Access to well-coordinated care should not be available only to those with the ability to pay. If high-quality primary care is a national goal, this sort of concierge service should be available to all. If insurance carriers offered concierge service as a part of their programs, they would likely discover that this type of coordinated care is more cost-effective than the fragmented care provided in typical managed care programs or fee-for-service care delivery systems.

Affordable comprehensive concierge care is available, but only to small numbers of patients. One example is the national program called the Program of All-Inclusive Care for the Elderly (PACE, described earlier), but this serves fewer than 20,000 patients and is generally restricted to very poor people who receive both Medicare- and Medicaid-financed health care and who have developed disabilities that would qualify them for nursing home placement. Other models are being developed, and the research necessary to justify their widespread dissemination continues. A valuable resource for effective innovative programs can be found at http://promisingpractices.fightchronicdisease.org; this site provides reliable brief summaries of programs that have been shown to work. You can enter your state into the website's search box to find programs that may be available in your area.

Our national political leaders and health care industry leaders—providers and insurers alike—must combine resources and focus their talents collectively on doing what is right for our nation's seniors. Solutions are available and more can and must be found. The health care crisis caused by the decreasing number of generalist physicians could not be solved by increasing the number of geriatricians to provide primary care for all U.S. seniors even if seniors were defined as only those over age 75; that is simply not possible, due to the small number (about 6,000) of geriatricians in the U.S. Rather, the solution is to be certain that all physicians, especially those training and practicing in the primary care disciplines of internal medicine and family medicine, are competent in geriatrics. That solution, in and of itself, will require tripling or quadrupling the number of geriatricians who currently serve as teachers, program developers, and researchers. Change is always difficult, but the crisis in health care has arrived and without urgent attention from all of us, it will certainly worsen.

6

Your Doctor's Perspective

Older people and their family members should understand something about the clinical approach and practice style of their generalist health care provider. You should be aware of what generally frames the physician's approach to your health care. Such an understanding will clarify your expectation of your doctor and his or her office staff. We believe that this knowledge of your physician and his or her practice will lead to a much better relationship between you and your doctor. What practice philosophy and character should you be on the lookout for during visits to your doctor?

Diagnosis

For most clinicians, seeing a patient for the first time is an engaging experience. The physician at once must come to know your medical situation while simultaneously establishing a relationship with you and often your family members. Ideally, the physician must demonstrate knowledge, communication skills, empathy, and compassion. You will want to be alert for such characteristics. Building a trusting relationship with you should be a rewarding experience for your doctor and the informed patient will sense whether the provider is engaged. Being invited to learn the intimate details of another person's life and circumstance leads to tight bonds. For the physician, "taking a history" from a patient is like reading a biography or experiencing a powerful character play or novel. It requires perception and sensitivity to understand the patient's concerns and to guide health care decisions that will resolve a problem or help a person better manage it.

The challenge for the physician is in the unknown aspects of you as a human being and the uncertainty of the problem or symptom. What is causing the symptom(s)? Is the source infection? Malignancy? Physical strain? Stress? Could it be a combination of factors? As primary care physicians, we both are dealing day in and day out with people who are worried about symptoms and health issues. Older persons characteristically bring extensive, lifelong experiences to their expectations regarding their health. We as clinicians must incorporate what we have learned of the patient's worldview and blend it with the mix of clinical issues at hand. The general physician must have a broad and deep understanding of disease, as well as interest in and compassion for the older person. With older patients, there is almost always a tension between the diagnosis or treatment of one problem and the possibility of causing a negative impact on another health problem that may or may not be known. These are the challenges the doctor faces, and because of them we have come to view the care of seniors as the most exciting and rewarding area of medicine.

Following you over years does not lessen your doctor's need for vigilance and good judgment. One of the greatest challenges for a primary care physician is detecting a new problem that slowly arises out of a cluster of chronic symptoms and conditions. For example, it is difficult to detect the emergence of the early signs of polymyalgia rheumatica (an inflammation of the soft tissues and joints) in a patient who has hypertension, diabetes, lung disease, and depression from the recent loss of a spouse. It is also difficult to present a new diagnosis to the patient without arousing undue fear. The doctor needs to share information with the patient but be sensitive to how much data you can take in at one time. It's a balancing act that when done successfully is as rewarding as any aspect of medicine.

For the primary care provider, learning to be watchful and alert to a patient's new health issues is fundamental and is different from when a patient arrives with symptoms of a single disease that requires diagnosis and treatment. In caring for older persons, the requirement for clinical judgment is paramount because of heterogeneity, multiple illnesses, and variable loss of physiological function, as discussed in Chapter 2. The primary care doctor uses judgment in arriving at a diagnosis, deciding on the pros and cons of laboratory tests or imaging studies. Always pursuing every symptom you discuss would create an unacceptable physical burden on you and potentially cause complications. Rather, expect your primary care provider to often use a strategy of careful watching, waiting, and worrying. The older and/or more vulnerable you are (or your ill relative is), the more important such a strategy becomes. For the same reasons, caution and good judgment are equally important in choosing treatment. An older person's body handles surgery and medicines differently from a middle-aged person's, and the presence of multiple diseases and variable physiological losses can mean that one treatment complicates another health problem or bodily function. You and your family members should expect such judgment and thoughtful reasoning.

A primary care physician may have to use diagnostically aggressive procedures with a senior, but this should never be done impulsively. Ordering an abdominal computed tomography (CT) scan with intravenous contrast for a 90-year-old patient who is frail and has kidney problems and heart failure is different from ordering such a procedure for an otherwise well 60-year-old. You should expect that your physician will involve you in decisions on diagnostic and treatment procedures, will tell you the consequences of any and all diagnostic and therapeutic options, and will educate you in clear and understandable terms about your clinical circumstances and the diagnostic and therapeutic choices available. A physician who meets these expectations exemplifies the fundamental role of the primary care physician as the patient's educator.

The practice of applying judgment and, when appropriate, taking the course of careful observation of a new health problem requires great responsibility on the part of your doctor. Many health care professionals argue that diagnostic caution and careful observation risk increased exposure to malpractice lawsuits. We argue the opposite: unexplained risks from diagnostic and therapeutic activities and recommendations lead to angry patients who are more likely to sue if a negative outcome occurs. On the other hand, a full explanation by your primary care provider of the possible consequences of any action or nonaction rarely results in litigation. In this day of multidisciplinary medical practice, such discussions and the rationale for each decision will be documented in the medical record. In fact, it has become our practice to dictate into the patient's medical record the content of the visit in the presence of the patient (and, when requested by the patient, also in the presence of those who have accompanied her or him). Patients have lauded such a practice as a way for them to further understand the facts and discussions related to the visit. You should insist on open and thorough discussions with your doctor.

Follow-up Visits

While you have the responsibility to communicate with your doctor about new symptoms or concerns, the burden should be on the physician or the primary care team to communicate with you about the follow-up of unsettled matters from a recent visit. This follow-up may be in reference to an unresolved symptom, laboratory evaluation, or imaging study. The responsibility for physicians to follow up should not be limited to primary care providers but applied to all clinicians, and it is already the practice of most physicians.

In our judgment, expecting the patient to initiate a call to follow up on some matter is risky, unreliable, and inconvenient for all. Most patients do not want to burden the physician with a follow-up call and will assume that not receiving a call from the physician or the physician's staff means that the test or study turned out fine. Such an assumption is dangerous, because a result or a laboratory evaluation or procedure may be abnormal but overlooked by the physician or lost in the shuffle of paper or electronic messages in a medical office. Most primary care physicians will have a system of follow-up communication with their patients. Some call the patients themselves, use e-mail, or send letters, and others assign the task to office staff. Most use a combination of these. Letting patients know the result of a test or imaging procedure relieves the worry of uncertainty that most patients feel. Further, it allows the physician or staff member to provide additional information and invites the patient to ask any questions about the results and questions that may have developed since the visit or that may have been forgotten during the visit, a common occurrence. Be sure that you understand how results will be communicated to you after each visit. The effective clinician's office will have established a system to be on the lookout for results of a procedure, such as a CT scan, in order to be certain that the procedure was performed and that the results have been transmitted. Some sort of reminder system that the physician and the staff have devised is important to avoid lost or misdirected reports.

Follow-up office visits are usually requested by the physician or his or her staff. In a primary care practice, well patients are usually seen yearly or every two years. But the older you are and/ or the more chronic illnesses you have, the more frequent your visits will be. The interval between scheduled visits will vary and depends on the judgment of your health care provider and on your input. A follow-up visit may be in one to seven days if a problem is not yet diagnosed, stabilized, or fully resolved. You should be certain about the timing of the follow-up and discuss this with the doctor before leaving the privacy of the examining room and proceeding to the checkout counter or desk. The receptionist should confirm your follow-up appointment as you leave.

House Calls

Performing a house call is a valuable service in primary care, and it is essential to delivering good-quality care for those who are homebound. Providing care at home for a senior who is bedbound is an act of respect and compassion. The inconvenience, discomfort, and stress involved in transporting someone who is homebound to an office or clinic for routine health care is not something that any of us would want for ourselves or a loved one.

There are great advantages for the physician in seeing you at home. The house call provides valuable insights about you and your support resources and teaches your doctor far more about your home situation than can be learned in an office environment. Upon entering your home, the physician can appreciate the following: something of your character and interests; what resources are at hand to provide support, if needed; what barriers exist to accomplishing clinical goals; whether you are able to do what is needed to maintain health and function while living at home; whether your home environment is safe or if fall risks (such as poor lighting or tripping hazards) are present. Your physician will get to know you much more deeply through a home visit. The better your doctor knows you, the more useful advice he or she can provide.

House calls can also lead to improved understanding and treatment of a patient's problem. Several examples follow:

- An 80-year-old woman developed numbness and pain in her legs. The problem remained unexplained even after an office evaluation and appropriate laboratory investigation. She had lived alone for years. She described eating a good diet and drinking one alcoholic beverage per day. Then one day, she fell, which prompted a house call. Her home was immaculate, and her fall seemed to have resulted from a stumble over a throw rug. In talking with her in the kitchen, one could easily notice in a partially opened cabinet several gallon bottles of whisky. Her one drink a day turned out to be a continuously replenished glass of whiskey, resulting in severe nerve damage. (A rotating group of friends obliged her regular requests to obtain whiskey every month, and each friend was led to believe that the supply was to last a year.)

- A patient who had frequent heart failure did not take her medications regularly; the house call revealed that she could not easily get down the stairs to the refrigerator, where they were kept.
- A man's kitchen was filled with chicken bones and unwashed dishes, and months of newspapers were unopened in the vestibule. His underlying dementia had been virtually undetectable when he came to the doctor's office twice a year for oversight of his hypertension, arthritis, visual impairment, and hearing disorder. He was brought to the office by an unsuspecting friend who waited for him at the curb, never seeing the inside of his home.
- A nearly 100-year-old woman who was living alone made a midwinter visit to an emergency department, was diagnosed with dehydration, and was instructed to increase her fluid intake. During a house call to the woman the next day, the source of the problem was recognized in minutes: the main water supply pipe to her home had frozen. She had a bottle of water but drank only a small amount each day because she was concerned that she would run out. Additionally, she had set the thermostat in her home to 92 degrees Fahrenheit, and the heat caused her to lose considerable water.

House calls are different from other kinds of encounters between doctors and patients. The fundamental role of the physician in all settings is to educate you about your health and how to optimize both health and functional ability. In your home, patient education is typically the primary focus of the visit. A physician has only rudimentary diagnostic tools that can be contained in the "black bag."

Unfortunately, however, relatively few physicians make house calls. Reasons typically given for this omission are inefficiency and relatively low reimbursement. Improving compensation for house calls would help, and this change should be a component of health care reform.

You should ask your primary care physician about his or her attitude toward performing house calls before there is any need for this service.

Learning from Patients

Among the greatest rewards of being a primary care physician, especially one who cares for older people, is the continual education we receive from patients. Older patients have a wealth of experiences, deep insights, and rich wisdom. Listening to them expands the world of the doctor.

In our practices, we have listened to stories of struggle, burdens, sadness, and challenges, as well as stories of joy and accomplishment. These first-hand patient narratives are the source of tremendous learning and a good dose of humility. Consider the following:

- the experiences of a man who had fought in the Battle of the Bulge, now feeling pain from a retained bullet
- the increasing isolation and depression of a 95-year-old mother after the death of her 70-year-old child
- the horror of a merchant mariner at having two of his transport ships sunk on the same day while attempting to supply material to Europe during World War II and now struggling with incapacitating ankle arthritis resulting from the fracture sustained when he had to jump 80 feet from the stern of the sinking vessel

- the stamina and dedication of a recently raped 86-year-old woman in overcoming the fear and apprehension of living alone
- the challenge and courage of a disabled 90-year-old father dealing with his 60-year-old son, who stole from him to buy illicit drugs
- the inner strength of an octogenarian to restore meaning and purpose to her life and overcome post-traumatic stress after being robbed and beaten to unconsciousness by an intruder after she had recently lost her husband of 60 years
- the development of the first cordless electric drill to be used in space exploration by a patient now struggling to deal with his ever-increasing infirmity and memory loss
- recurring nightmares about the landings of D-Day in one who participated in those many years ago
- the courage of a nonagenarian without family, friends, or resources facing terminal cancer
- the insights of a government official who had struggled to determine policy to bring the war in Vietnam to an end, now becoming bedbound from multiple vertebral fractures
- the commitment of an 85-year-old great-grandmother to care for an abandoned 12-year-old great-grandchild despite her own physical disabilities

The primary care provider who has gotten to know an individual over many years has more opportunity to develop the trust required for a patient to share such experiences. Patients of any age can teach the empathetic and astute physician about the meaning and purpose of life, but seniors, because of their longer experience, more often have powerful stories to share. The health care provider who is willing to listen to your stories, even when told in serial format, will more definitively understand your life and be better able to advise you.

You teach your primary care provider in another important way: you teach about medicine. Most physicians understand that their patients are their best teachers. You can sense this attitude on the part of your physician by his or her expression of interest and by how carefully the doctor attends to the details of the story you share.

Each patient makes the thoughtful and inquiring doctor a better physician. It has amazed us how much a patient can teach simply by coming to see us with a new complaint or issue. The physician's simple question, "What do you think may be wrong?" almost always yields meaningful clues about the patient's central need. Patients often have insights about developing symptoms that can help guide the doctor. Asking your opinion about new symptoms is a sign of respect, good judgment, insight, and humility on the part of your physician.

7

Getting the Most from Your Referral to a Specialist

Y ou and your family should have some understanding of
the professional relationship that your generalist physician and a specialist have with each other in order to
maximize the benefit of your visit to that specialist. A few basic
points about the different roles and approaches of the generalist
and the specialist will help you know what to expect.

The Difference between a Consultant Specialist and a Primary Care Provider

The role of the consultant specialist (physician or surgeon) in outpatient practice is different from the role of a generalist (primary
care physician). First, the consultant needs to address a specific
question or series of questions. If the referring physician or the
patient does not word the question(s) clearly, the consultant will

need to communicate with the referring physician's office and talk with the patient and in many instances the patient's family. Here are examples of patients' opening questions or statements when seeing a consultant:

- What is causing this chest pain?
- What should I do to control my recently diagnosed rheumatoid arthritis?
- Do I need surgery for my continuing back pain?
- My doctor thinks I may have an endocrine problem.

Compare these with the possible starting points of the same patients with a generalist:

- I have pain under my breastbone when lifting my 2-year-old granddaughter.
- I feel tired and stiff in the morning.
- My back aches after playing tennis.
- I am losing hair and have no energy.

The generalist must consider a broader explanation, that several problems may be emerging in proximity, or the onset of new symptoms in the presence of existing chronic health problems.

Second, from the consultant's perspective, there is generally greater pressure to establish a diagnosis quickly. After all, a patient who comes to a specialist or subspecialist, whether self-referred or referred by another physician, is expecting an answer. The typical consultant approach of urgently establishing a diagnosis may lead to the early initiation of diagnostic efforts. While this approach is often appropriate, it may also have negative consequences: the patient may become anxious; an unrelated abnormality may be found that is not significant; or injury to the patient may occur from a diagnostic test or procedure. In addition, health care costs will go up.

The generalist physician's approach of "watching, waiting, and worrying" when initial symptoms are not well defined is appropriate when the patient is in no imminent danger. The physician must be reassuring and comforting to the patient while also mindful that the clinical course is not yet defined and close surveillance is necessary. It is incumbent on the specialist physician to recognize this difference in approach and, when appropriate, to take an observational approach as well. This is especially true for older patients, who are at increased risk of problems caused by diagnostic or therapeutic interventions. Older patients typically have multiple chronic health problems; therefore, focusing on just one problem, as sometimes occurs with a specialist, may lead to a diagnostic procedure or treatment that could exacerbate a separate condition.

The ideal consulting specialist explains to the patient his or her thinking and approach to diagnosis and/or treatment. A plan to initiate a diagnostic approach in a week or two if symptoms intensify, expand, or fail to decrease can be a thoughtful way to proceed with older persons. But without good communication, this approach could lead the patient to be angry and resentful if a serious diagnosis is later established.

In the "watch, wait, and worry" approach, the generalist or specialist must be attentive and alert to any evolution of symptoms. It is the physician's responsibility to follow the patient closely with repeat visits, physician-initiated phone calls, or other means of communication. It is not adequate or even appropriate for the physician simply to leave the follow-up burden with the patient by saying, "Call me" if symptoms change, worsen, or fail to resolve. Patients often do not want to disturb the physician and may not report a subtle change in symptoms.

We both were specialists before becoming generalists. Understanding the perspective of a primary care physician would have made us better consultants.

A referral to a specialist may have been initiated in order for the specialist to perform a procedure, but often the generalist is also hoping for judgment, wisdom, sage advice, and help. This is especially true when the patient is older and has several health problems and vulnerabilities. Unfortunately, many specialists respond to a referring physician's request for a consultation with a long list of diagnostic possibilities, laboratory results, and possible procedures to determine the precise cause of a problem. This can be wasteful and confusing and is often unhelpful.

Qualities of an Ideal Consultation

Before an ideal consultation may be held, it is the generalist's responsibility to describe the patient's background to the consultant and to frame the question or questions that the specialist should address. This need not take much time and can be done by means of a letter, e-mail, or telephone call. In complicated situations, a phone call is often easiest. If the consultant is not available to receive a call, then communication by the generalist with a member of the specialist's staff usually is satisfactory.

Below we describe several qualities of effective and ideal consultations. With these in mind, you and your family members will be better able to evaluate the effectiveness of a consultation.

Good communication. You should expect that the consulting specialist will communicate promptly with your referring physician. Depending on the problem and the urgency, this communication may be by a phone call followed by a letter, by e-mail followed by letter, or by letter alone. Unless the consultant works regularly with a small and totally reliable and punctual administrative staff, it is usually not satisfactory for the consultant to write a note or dictate a summary and then expect it to be sent to your physician. Too often, delays or lapses at any of a number of levels make this form of communication inadequate. This happens particularly in academic environments, where specialists may be distracted by other responsibilities, whether teaching, committee work, administration, and/or research. The practice of simply putting a note in a large paper chart and assuming that the primary care physician will find it in a timely manner is unacceptable in most systems. Entering a note in an electronic record that is readable by the generalist may avoid the problem, but your referring physician should generally be alerted to the presence of such a note. The communication should be succinct and pithy and not repeat the material that your doctor had sent the consultant. The emphasis should be on the consultant's thinking and suggestions, and the specific diagnosis or results and treatment suggestions should be clearly worded. Occasionally, a consultant and your primary care doctor hold different opinions; in this situation, communication between the two physicians is especially critical. Also, new symptoms or signs may have developed while you were waiting to see a consultant, and these are best discussed with your doctor immediately.

Accessibility and punctuality. Ideally, a physician consultant (or his or her associate) is available for urgent as well as routine consultations. Waits of more than three weeks are often frustrating to you as well as to your referring physician. The very act of deciding to request a consultation creates concern and apprehension for you. Prolonged waits worsen these feelings and may lead to an initially poor relationship between you and the consultant. In addition, the problem needing attention may progress. Most consultants have developed strategies to keep wait times reasonably short. Such strategies include offering an extra appointment slot as needed or, if demand remains high, recruiting an associate.

Thoughtfulness. The ideal consultant is thoughtful and focused on you and your unique situation. In geriatrics, where often there are many confounding issues, this characteristic is mandatory. Occasionally, some consultants "miss the forest for the trees" when encountering a patient who has many problems. Using a clinical textbook approach is something a generalist can do and is generally not helpful for a consultant to record in the report. Rather, your generalist provider is seeking judgment targeted to your unique issues, not a textbook reiteration. One of our colleagues has often referred to this issue of consultant thoughtfulness as a partnership of consultant and generalist. This colleague would argue that for patients with complex problems he seeks a thoughtful deliberation rather than an opinion.

Focus. The consultant physician should answer the question(s) posed by your physician when the consultation is requested. Your physician should initiate the consultation with a clear question or questions to be answered. If such a question is not stated, then the wise consultant will phone your doctor to discern the reason for the request. If the generalist is not available, usually the office staff can decipher the reason by looking through the patient's chart. The wise consultant will ask you for your expectation of the consultation, even if your primary care doctor had already stated one. When these requests diverge, as they often do, the consultant should address your concerns and those of your doctor as well. Nothing is more frustrating for your referring physician than receiving a written consultation that doesn't address the core questions. Likewise, nothing is more frustrating for the consultant than seeing a patient without any stated reason for the request. For you as the patient, nothing is more frustrating than to have made the long-awaited visit to a specialist and then to leave the office with questions not fully answered.

Practicality. The ideal consultant will give you and your doctor practical advice as to next steps: what action should take place and by whom, when, and how. Examples include precise doses of recommended medications, side effects to look out for, how best and how often a patient given a new medication is to be monitored, and what adjustments to the medication or dosage might be needed. When a procedure is completed, your doctor needs to know when the results will be available and that the consultant will analyze them and review the results with him or her. Occasionally, a new or unexpected problem is identified. If this is the case, the consultant should describe the expected course of the problem and how the outcome may be altered with any treatment.

Humility. Almost all patients we have referred for consultation report back on the nature of the visit. Sometimes this report is by phone, but typically it is a point of discussion at the next scheduled appointment with your primary care doctor. The advice provided is discussed, but so is the demeanor of the consultant and his or her staff. If anyone was less than courteous, this may be described. A consultant's warmth and concern are invariably appreciated. When you report to your doctor that the consultant displayed arrogance, disrespect, or curtness, then he or she knows the consultation will be of little or no value. Most patients judge the entire staff, but all too often the problem is with the consultant rather than the rest of the staff. On rare occasions, a consultant fails to respect the relationship you have with your doctor. The patient's perception of the relationship with the generalist is paramount, and the specialist is the invited guest. Especially in situations in which a consultant believes your primary doctor has made an error or shown poor judgment, the consultant should talk with the referring physician to understand her or his thinking. Only by doing this can a truly effective consultation be accomplished. Sometimes, you may find that a consultant is judgmental about your doctor, even though they see the patient at a later time, perhaps with more information, and with no idea of the complex situation that prevailed when the consultation was requested. Criticism of the generalist often leads to distrust of the consultant and may fracture any effective relationship between the two physicians or between you and either physician. There is no place for arrogance in medicine. When a consultant feels that your generalist is off base, you should expect that the two physicians will talk promptly.

Referral for a Specific Procedure

When you are referred specifically for a diagnostic procedure, your referring physician's general assumption is that the procedure will be scheduled and performed, with feedback provided soon after. When the specialist thinks that such a procedure is inappropriate, she or he should discuss this concern with the referring physician. Likewise, if additional or different procedures are recommended, it is imperative that the consultant communicate with your referring physician before moving forward, with the obvious exception of situations in which the consultant deems life-saving measures to be required. All too often, a patient calls their primary care provider about symptoms that have developed after a procedure or calls about the results of a procedure of which the generalist has no knowledge. This leads to confusion and inadequate health care. The consultant should inform the generalist's office whenever she or he performs a procedure, especially if the generalist did not know the procedure was planned. When the consultant is not certain what options are best diagnostically or therapeutically, it is best to confer with your referring physician, who has a deeper understanding of the full situation. In our experience, such communication is invariably helpful to both practitioners.

Further Work-up, Further Consultation, and Follow-up

A specialist will usually communicate with the referring physician before proceeding with any invasive work-up (unless such work-up was specified as the reason for the referral). The same holds true for further referral of the patient to another specialist. Patients often call the generalist physician to ask about the results of a consultation. If the generalist is unaware of what has transpired, then the patient may feel angry, disrespected, and confused. Except in emergency or urgent situations, this should never happen. On too many occasions, we have been called when a patient has a complication after a procedure or an ill effect from a medicine prescribed by a consultant, and we were not aware of the procedure or the medicine. Patient care is compromised in this situation. Furthermore, the generalist may have had good reason to avoid a procedure or a specific medicine. The ideal consultant will respect that concern and at least consider and discuss it with the referring generalist. Communication these days is easy by e-mail, phone, or facsimile, so physicians should never fail to convey information. Once we have a universal, patient-specific, and transportable electronic patient record system, many of these sorts of communication problems will disappear, but that day has not yet arrived.

Recently, an 85-year-old woman came in to the office because of diarrhea and dizziness. She said it had started about 10 days after a visit to an otolaryngologist to whom she was referred because of diminishing hearing. What she did not report was that she had been given a one-week course of an antibiotic by the consulting physician for treatment of a suspected sinus infection. She didn't connect the onset of the diarrhea to taking the antibiotic and didn't mention taking it. Neither a written nor verbal consultation report had arrived in the office by the time she was seen, so it was uncertain what had been done by the consultant. Only after a review of drugs she had recently taken did her recent use of an antibiotic come to light. Indeed, she had developed a serious antibiotic-associated diarrheal illness that took over six weeks to fully resolve.

Your follow-up after the initial consultation is best worked out between the specialist and your referring generalist. What will be done, when, and by whom are all critical issues that a consultant should discuss with you and your primary care provider. The consultant, in our judgment, should not assume an ongoing co-management arrangement. Co-management may be appropriate in certain situations, but it is overdone to some extent and can lead to confusion for the patient and to prescriptions and recommendations that work at cross-purposes to what the generalist is trying to accomplish. Older individuals often find it physically difficult to get to a physician's office, and seeing more than one physician on an ongoing basis may be a burden. It also increases costs.

Some generalists will want to involve a specialist on an ongoing basis, but this is something that you, the specialist, and your generalist should decide together to avoid confusion and redundancy. This practice of co-management occurs frequently, especially after a patient is hospitalized and consultants have seen the patient in the hospital and scheduled a follow-up appointment. With the popularity of hospitalists, who care for patients only in the hospital and may be disconnected from the patient's primary care provider, the practice of obtaining multiple consultations with subsequent scheduled specialist follow-up is common. The office-based generalist in this situation may have difficulty sorting out who is doing what, when, and why. Patients often find that contacting their generalist is simpler than contacting a specialist and so naturally call their generalist with any concerns.

On many occasions, each of us has been called by a patient asking about possible side effects or the rationale for a new medication prescribed by a consultant and we have no idea what the medication is or the rationale for giving it. Not having up-to-date information puts the generalist at a disadvantage and compromises your health care.

A consultant physician will occasionally make a follow-up appointment for a patient when the main reason is the physician's own interest. While understandable and perhaps laudable, this practice creates an expensive and inconvenient situation for the patient. A consultant physician can often follow up by asking the primary care physician how a patient is doing. Some consultants, most notably surgeons, oncologists, and therapeutic radiologists, do this by mailing the primary care physician a simple form to be completed and returned on a periodic or occasional basis.

When You or Your Family Requests a Consultation

At times, a patient may initiate a consultation without a generalist's involvement. The patient may not *have* a generalist or may decide to self-refer without communicating with the primary care provider. We don't encourage this, as it leads to fragmentation of an individual's health care and less than ideal medical practice. A consultation generated in this way is often more difficult because it must start from scratch rather than follow a previsit communication about the patient's needs and the clinical reason for the referral. Most generalists are not threatened when a patient or family member asks about obtaining a consultation. Resisting such a request is usually divisive and ill advised. The wise generalist will welcome the opportunity for a second opinion and work with the consultant to frame the issues clearly.

In managed care environments, the patient-generated request for consultation is common. The reasons that many administrators have resisted allowing patients direct and easy access to consultants include cost control and protection of specialist time for conditions that require specialist care. In geriatrics, when patient-generated requests for consultation occur, it seems to us that it is the generalist's responsibility to discuss with the patient (and/or family) the pros and cons of such consultation and then mutually decide on the best course of action. Often when a physician's judgment is compromised by a financial conflict of interest, the patient is not well served. For example, the physician may have aggregate financial risk for the expense of consultation in some managed care situations; in this situation, a physician's strong resistance to a requested consultation will sow patient dissatisfaction and distrust.

The Consultant as Teacher

Fundamentally, physicians are educators. For doctors who do not perform medical procedures, teaching patients and their families is the core of their responsibility, and most do this well. Also, the best consultants we have worked with do this routinely and carefully document their conversations with patients and family members. They also take time to teach the referring physician by providing a brief update of current literature and the evidence basis for the consultant's thoughts and recommendation. Such notes are valuable to the generalist and lead to specific, case-based learning, which may be the most effective and efficient method for a health care provider to stay up to date. The educational component of a consultation need not be long and indeed it is best when it is pithy and includes reference to a relevant article from the medical literature that the generalist can easily access. Consultation notes of this nature, while not common, reflect the work of top-tier consultants.

8

Geriatrics Education for All Health Care Providers

The chance that you can find a physician with formal training in geriatrics is slim. The heart of the problem is the dearth of medical education provided to students and postgraduate trainees about the unique health issues and needs of seniors. Indeed, even with the obvious dramatic increase in the number of older adults in the United States in recent decades, there persists a serious mismatch between the content of medical education and the health care needs of the population. This mismatch in professional education will affect nearly every senior who seeks excellent health care. Being informed about the origins of this health care workforce shortage and understanding current efforts to rectify the problem will help you find the best care for yourself.

The remarkable increase in the number of seniors in the United States and all other developed countries is well known and is commonly referred to as a "demographic imperative."

Life expectancy has risen approximately 30 years since the beginning of the twentieth century and now approaches age 80. In the United States, the aging of the baby boomers (members of the larger-than-usual cohort born during the 15 years after World War II) will markedly expand the number of seniors. The oldest baby boomers will reach age 65 in 2010. By the year 2030 they will have swelled the ranks of those age 65 or older to 78 million, approximately 23 percent of the population. The impact of this demographic imperative will be widespread and will profoundly affect the costs and delivery of health care.

Seniors make heavy use of the health care system. Currently, seniors constitute about 15 percent of the population but are responsible for nearly 50 percent of health care expenditures. Except for pediatricians and obstetricians, nearly all physicians see older patients. Seniors make up one-third to two-thirds of the patients in the practices of many specialists (including urology, orthopedic surgery, and ophthalmology) and subspecialists (including cardiology, endocrinology, and gastroenterology). The practice of generalist physicians (general internal medicine, family medicine, and geriatric medicine) is typically dominated by seniors. These proportions will increase rapidly with the aging of the baby boomers.

The difficulty this presents for your health care is related to the current educational priorities of health professional schools in the United States. Although there were a few pioneers in geriatrics beginning around the middle of the last century, most physicians who finished medical school or postgraduate training before the mid-1980s received no training in geriatrics at all. It was not until the mid-1980s that a few medical educators introduced the topic. Several major philanthropic organizations, such as the John A. Hartford Foundation, Atlantic Philanthropies, and the Donald W. Reynolds Foundation, fundamentally changed this deficiency in U.S. medical education by providing grants to medical, nursing, social work, and other health care professional schools to develop programs in geriatrics. This effort has been sustained and has increased over the years, leading to a major enhancement of medical education in geriatrics in the United States. Despite these efforts, which have entailed the investment of several hundred million dollars in U.S. medical education, there remains much to do. Many medical schools and postgraduate training programs still offer little or no training in geriatrics, and too few graduates are trained adequately in the unique problems of seniors.

There are some exceptions, and models do exist for large-scale training of professionals in geriatric medicine. The Veterans Affairs (VA) Medical Centers have long emphasized training and research in geriatrics, and in those schools that have a relationship with a VA medical center, students and trainees have had some good exposure to geriatrics. Recently, the federal government (in addition to the VA) has put some effort into geriatrics training. The Health Resources and Services Administration (HRSA) has offered competitive grants to improve and expand geriatrics education for health care professionals. The difficulty with the HRSA initiative is that little funding (approximately $31 million in FY 2009 for the entire country) is allocated to these programs relative to the need.

The shortage of geriatricians is the thesis of an Institute of Medicine report released in 2008, "Retooling for an Aging America: Building the Health Care Workforce" (available from the National Academies Press). In this report, health care professionals are described as "too small [in number] and woefully unprepared" to meet the needs of U.S. seniors. Important corroborating data have been collected since 2000 by the University of Cincinnati's Institute for the Study of Health: the ADGAP (Association of Directors of Geriatric Academic Programs) Status of Geriatrics Workforce Study has tracked the number of geriatricians in practice and in academic programs over the years. These data report that fewer than 300 physicians enter a formal postgraduate training program in geriatric medicine in the United States each year. About half of those entering programs to receive geriatrics training graduated from medical schools outside the U.S., a reflection of the unpopularity of the field in American medical schools. In 2007, fewer physicians entered training for a career in geriatrics than at any time in the last 10 years. The number of geriatric medicine trainees in the United States entering a second or third year of training fell to less than 40 individuals in 2007. In addition to shortages in clinical practice and education, this problem results in a dearth of physician scientists trained to do the much-needed research that will result in new knowledge aimed at improving the health care of seniors.

Such deficiencies in education may result in the failure of specialists to provide the highest-quality care for their oldest patients. Examples of this are the failure to recognize postoperative delirium in an older patient, leading to a fall and further complications; uncertainty in knowing how to weigh the risks of surgery for a senior; not realizing the dangers and adverse effects of using certain drugs for seniors; refusing to perform surgery on the basis of age alone; and lack of awareness of the need for older postoperative patients to become mobile soon after a procedure.

The lead taken by private philanthropic organizations in addressing this deficiency in medical education and research is one reason for optimism. As of January 2010, one such program, the Dennis W. Jahnigen Career Development Scholars Award Program, had supported 79 surgical or surgery-related medical specialists in committing their careers to the geriatric aspects of their specialty. These awards have been funded by the John A. Hartford Foundation, Atlantic Philanthropies, and the grantees' own institutions. Through these career development awards, physicians are supported early in their careers to develop approaches that will foster improvements in the care of older patients. The goal is to increase understanding of the unique challenges posed by older patients. It is hoped and expected that these physician-scholars will advocate within their specialty organizations for more teaching and research in geriatrics.

The vision behind this educational approach was to encourage practitioners in surgery-related medical disciplines to focus on the care of seniors needing surgery. This focus would begin from the moment a patient is admitted to a hospital and continue through postoperative rehabilitation. These awards are available to physicians from the disciplines of emergency medicine, anesthesiology, general surgery, gynecology, otolaryngology, orthopedic surgery, ophthalmology, thoracic surgery, urology, and physical therapy and rehabilitation. When additional funds can be found, training may expand to other specialties, such as neurosurgery, radiology, dermatology, and others. This program for specialists and surgical subspecialties has provided a template for geriatrics training. Perhaps unique in U.S. medicine, this multidisciplinary training program is the product of the altruistic collaboration of leaders from 10 different medical specialties who have come together to focus on improving the health care of seniors. Building on programs that have supported the development of new knowledge, a second type of program has been designed to develop curricula to teach geriatrics to specialty trainees. While the number of such grants is relatively small compared to the need, it is a start, and it creates a model for other programs to follow.

From these beginnings, a research agenda has been developed. This work has inspired books on geriatric principles, and annual scientific meetings have been instituted that feature improvement of health care for seniors in the 10 participating specialties. A similar program, the T. Franklin Williams Scholars Program, also funded by the John A. Hartford Foundation and Atlantic Philanthropies, in partnership with subspecialty organizations, provides two-year awards to young physician investigators who have finished training in the subspecialties of internal medicine, such as cardiology, gastroenterology, and nephrology. This program may serve as a template for other initiatives. Through a wide variety of programs, the Department of Veterans Affairs has supported the development of many academic leaders with expertise in geriatrics. Finally, the Paul B. Beeson Career Development Award Program, which funds a variety of specialists, was originally supported only by foundations; now, due to its great success in training academic leaders with expertise in geriatrics, it has been expanded through joint funding from foundations, the subspecialty societies, and the NIH.

All of these major efforts, while vitally important, are only a start in meeting the need for more geriatrics training of the U.S. health care workforce. To have the needed impact, such initiatives must be adopted by the American Association of Medical Colleges and the postgraduate specialty training councils and be supported through specified funding from the Centers for Medicare and Medicaid Services, the current funder of the majority of postgraduate medical education in the United States.

In dealing with this situation, you can be comforted by awareness of a fundamental precept: even after their formal training, health care professionals learn from their practice and from their patients. Indeed, the continuing evolution of a health care provider's knowledge is derived from personal experience and continued learning. So today, there are many health care providers perfectly able to meet your needs who never received formal training in geriatrics but have learned the discipline through practice and experience. This book is designed to help you recognize such individuals and to develop an ideal relationship with them.

Faced with this demographic imperative and to date, the relatively meager governmental response, what is your role? First, be aware of the relatively small number of geriatricians in the United States. Second, be aware of the efforts to remedy the situation. Third, work through national organizations such as the Foundation for Health in Aging of the American Geriatrics Society (www.americangeriatrics.org), AARP (www.aarp.org), and others to effect a change in the profile of the health care workforce. It is likely to be the outcry of citizens to our national leaders and politicians that ultimately will bring the reform that is needed. Such reform must fully awaken our health care systems and professional schools to the crisis in primary care for seniors. This can occur only through enhanced research and education and by modifying our Medicare program so that it will offer incentives to young professionals to choose a career serving older people.

Managing Your Health

9

How to Take Charge

Americans are achieving historic longevity. In fact, many of us can anticipate spending about one-third of our lifetime as senior citizens. Despite this optimistic news, we generally have not embraced the concept of self-responsibility for our health. In fact, most of us devote far less time to planning and managing our health than to planning and managing our vacations. For the oldest of us, this neglect is perhaps understandable, because we grew up in an era when health decisions were the purview of physicians (the majority of whom never received any formal or even informal training in geriatrics). But for the baby boom population now beginning to reach eligibility for Medicare, these passive attitudes need reform.

Let us summarize the take-charge principles we like to share with our patients:

We are each ultimately responsible for our own decisions regarding health. This is equally true whether we carry the burden of chronic illness or have been fortunate enough to be in excellent health.

Get the best medical care you can. Find a primary care physician who is knowledgeable about the aging process. This may be your most important health-related decision. He or she should have excellent listening skills and have similarly skilled associates. Increasingly, health care leaders are exploring the concept of a "Medical Home" (discussed earlier). Such a concept would require reconfiguration of primary care practices so that some will serve as a safe haven for seniors for navigating the complex health care system. If you have been with your personal physician for decades, he or she may be thinking of retiring and might be glad to discuss with you a transition to a younger physician. Better to do this before you find yourself acutely ill and with no primary care doctor who knows you and your values. Most physicians who are planning to leave practice will raise this fact with you and make suggestions for finding a new health care provider. The hospitals with which your medical group affiliates should value older patients and provide some or all of the supportive services that you may someday need, such as rehabilitation, home health care, social workers, and access to specialist physicians with interest in and knowledge of the special needs of seniors. In choosing a doctor, focus on the values you feel are most critical in your generalist. A commonly used expression makes this point: "Do not let perfection be the enemy of the good." Above all, make sure your generalist has empathy and compassion and is a good communicator and an attentive listener. There are many sources of information about physicians, but the best source remains word of mouth from patients.

Understand your illnesses and conditions and be an active participant in key decisions. There are abundant and easily accessible sources of information about the aging process and the diseases experienced more commonly in older age. While your first and primary source should be your personal health care provider, the Internet can be of enormous help. We recommend the excellent health and wellness website created for older adults by the National Institutes of Health (www.NIHSeniorHealth.gov). Take notes, write down questions, and bring them to your next visit to your primary care provider.

Know your medications. Powerful medications can have powerful side effects, and overmedication is a constant concern in geriatrics. When we ask our patients what medicines they are taking (and this should happen at every visit), we are fearful when a patient talks about the "blue oblong pill" or the "little yellow one." Such vagaries are their own "prescription for disaster." Have your health care professional's staff write down the names of your medications, and ask what each of these drugs does and what the common side effects are. Your pharmacist can also help in this regard. If the descriptions from the drugstore are in small print, then ask the pharmacist or pharmacy assistant to explain the information. We have long promoted the "shopping bag" test of simply emptying your medicine cabinet into a convenient bag and bringing the whole collection to your doctor's office. Be sure to include any nonprescription medications, especially those used as cold or allergy remedies. Do not omit vitamins and minerals and your favorite alternative medicines, such as herbal supplements. In our experience, by the time you and your health care provider are finished going through this collection of medicines, you will have a lighter bag to take home. There are excellent sources of information on prescription drugs, side effects, and interactions with other drugs at the National Institutes of Health website cited above.

Keep accurate health records. If you have ever browsed through a used book store, you may have run across family Bibles with the equivalent of copious health records of family members written in the margins. The modern version of this practice is the personal health record. Until all records are available electronically, a simple notebook will suffice. Record the following essential information:

- A signed copy of your advance health directive and the name, phone number, and address of your surrogate decision maker, if you have one. States vary in the terms of requirements for these advance directives, but the most important element is to have selected a trusted surrogate and alternate decision maker to speak for you if you are unable. Also be certain that you share your ideas about your health care and the use or nonuse of life-supportive strategies in case you experience a catastrophic event such as a massive heart attack or stroke.
- An updated list of all medications, including doses and the frequency with which you take them.
- Updated blood pressure and body weight determinations.
- Any laboratory test result (such as hemoglobin A1C, a marker of sugar control in diabetes) that is being followed regularly.
- The names and phone numbers of all your active health care providers.

Make smart lifestyle decisions. By all means, follow a prudent life style, the "big three" elements of which are: weight management, physical exercise, and continued mental and social stimulation.

Obesity is becoming perhaps the most important health issue for many Americans, with the exception of the very oldest. Everyone should know his or her body mass index (BMI) and seek nutritional advice if obese. The BMI can easily be calculated from your weight and height. Simply enter "BMI" in your web-based search engine, and one or several published formulas and information to interpret the result will appear. Being heavy puts strain on joints, and excessive body fat promotes higher levels of inflammation in the body and is harmful to the cardiovascular system, the metabolic regulators, and certain aspects of brain function.

Regular physical exercise is perhaps the single factor that can improve and sustain the highest possible level of functioning in older age. In addition to the positive effect exercise has on muscular function, strength, and balance, there is emerging evidence that moderate regular exercise promotes brain function, especially memory.

Humans are inherently social beings. Survey studies have found that loneliness and isolation, which are common in later life, are associated with a deterioration of mental function and with acceleration of the severity of many chronic disease states. Hard as it is at times for seniors who have lost many lifelong friends, it is important to seek out companions through senior centers, religious groups, neighborhoods, and other organized and informal community activities.

10

How to Choose a Doctor and Make the Most of Your Appointment

Finding a Primary Care Physician

You face a challenge in finding a suitable primary care physician. Even if you already have a longstanding, comfortable relationship with a generalist physician and have no plans to move, doctors retire, curtail their practices, and die. If you find yourself in such a situation, a few pointers can help.

If you are seeking a new physician in your home area, ask for recommendations from friends, family members, and doctors in your community. This is the starting point for most people. If you are in a managed care program or are participating in certain insurance programs, the company will provide you with a list of physicians who are accepting new patients. These doctors have met certain quality standards. All county medical societies maintain a physician referral program. If you use this service, be sure to find out whether the recommended physicians accept Medicare.

We mentioned earlier that various types of doctors (family physicians, internists, geriatricians) are especially qualified to provide primary care. Current board certification is a common standard of quality, and you should feel free to ask the physician's office staff if the physician is board certified. You can usually obtain the same information from various websites.

Other factors you may want to consider are location and solo versus group practice. The location of the primary office is often especially important for seniors, as is access to parking and public transportation. There are few solo practitioners these days, and all physicians have to have a system of coverage when they are unavailable during emergencies and vacations. Find out who covers for your doctor during absences and, if it is a group practice, who the other physicians in the group are.

Interacting with the Physician

A positive, nurturing relationship with a primary care physician can be one of the most important factors in maintaining good health. Sadly, both patients and physicians often report that their interactions leave something to be desired. Patients complain that it is difficult to schedule appointments promptly, that there are long waits in the office, and that contact time with their often-distracted doctor is too brief. Primary care physicians complain that their schedules are too crowded, that health maintenance organizations (HMOs) limit the time allowed for each patient visit, that paperwork is endless, and that prescription renewal and drug plan requests take too long.

We optimistically await major reform in the health care system that will make satisfying visits to a health care provider the norm. However, even in today's constrained environment in primary health care, both the patient and the physician can take steps to enhance the office visit. This will help doctors and other primary care providers exercise the aim of our profession: individual, attentive, compassionate, and comprehensive care of the patient. For good intentions to be turned into the best possible medical care, we must have a set of mutual assumptions and a "Patient-Physician Bill of Rights," so to speak. Knowing these principles will help you in every encounter with a health care professional, especially your primary care provider.

The patient has the right to a personal physician's full attention, the right to courteous and individualized care, the right to express health concerns and obtain answers, and the right to the assurance that promises made will be honored and that any unsettled issue will be resolved. The health care provider is responsible for seeing that every medical encounter reaches closure (that is, the patient is informed of conclusions and understands the plan of diagnosis or treatment being suggested). The patient is responsible for being considerate of the time pressures of the physician, for following advice, and for knowledge of medications and health practices unique to his or her individualized care. Both the health care provider and the patient have the right to be treated with courtesy and respect by each other.

Attitudes may lead to communication problems. Many of the current older generation tend to be deeply respectful of authority figures and may need prompting to fully describe their reasons for seeking medical attention. It is to be hoped that ageist attitudes—the negative prejudgment of seniors—are rare in health care professionals. If you encounter ageism, be leery of the ability of that professional to provide ideal care to older patients. Additionally, many health care professionals may find it difficult to shift from a disease-specific orientation to an assessment-of-function approach, which should be the cornerstone of a successful encounter with an older patient. Older persons are concerned about the real, and imagined, impacts of normal aging and of age-related diseases on their ability to independently carry out the activities of daily life. The health care provider, through his or her recommendations and treatments, can support and improve, or take away, elements of that independence.

This all seems straightforward, but what can we do to facilitate the implementation of these mutual rights and responsibilities? Let's start with what you can do as a patient to maximize your visits to the doctor.

A Successful Office Visit

After decades of relating to older patients and their caregivers, we have developed strategies that help us maximize available time, resulting in a more satisfying office visit for both our patients and for us.

Make a List of Your Concerns. Probably the most important thing you can do to improve your visit is to write down any issues you want to discuss. Plan the list well before the day of the visit, and review it carefully. It's your health, so raise any matter of concern to you. There is no inappropriate, silly, or trivial issue. If it is important to you, it should be important to your health care provider. Don't prejudge what is important or not. Before reading the items or presenting the list to your doctor, consider starting with the *last* item on the list. Typically, that last item will have the most personal significance to you. We've found that a typical list might read:

Postnasal drip
Trouble sleeping
Indigestion
I think I have cancer

Ideally, the time that you are talking should consume about half of the visit. If your health care provider does the majority of the talking, then your concerns will not be dealt with fully. Be sure that you understand the information you are given and that all of your concerns have been discussed.

Mention Any Limitations. A growing literature suggests that in the busy office setting, there may be significant barriers to communication that are attributable to the patient and/or the physician. Older patients often have limitations of function in sight and hearing, physical functioning, and cognition. At the time of the first visit, if the physician is unaware of these barriers to communication, precious time is lost, and the potential for misinterpretation of information in a time-pressured environment is great. Therefore, at the start of a visit, make known any such limitations you have; they are nothing to be embarrassed about.

Know Your Medications. By law, pharmacies provide detailed information to you every time you fill a prescription. Therefore, it is easy to identify a medicine by name and know its strength. However, the information pharmacies provide is typically exhaustive, hard to interpret, and sometimes frightening, so many people do not read it closely. You should find out from your doctor (or from less intimidating reading material provided by your doctor) why the medication was prescribed and what common side effects you might experience. Don't forget to include nonprescription medications in the list you report to your doctor. If you have any doubts, pack all your medications and other health-related substances (such as vitamins) into a bag and bring them to the office visit. This is an especially good idea for your first visit with a new health care provider.

Don't Mislead Your Doctor or Minimize Your Concerns. At times, we may be embarrassed about certain concerns or reluctant to admit that we have not followed recommendations. Misleading or incomplete information can cause a medical error. No matter how embarrassing you may consider the information, rest assured that your doctor will treat you with respect and will maintain confidentiality. (Also rest assured that your doctor has heard it many times before.)

Explain Your Values. If your doctor does not ask, share your cultural and religious values regarding medical treatment and end-of-life issues. These are important to medical decision making. In particular, it is mandatory to have discussions with your primary care physician regarding end-of-life decisions. We are all aware that with the many advances in medicine, prolongation of biological life is not always synonymous with a good-quality existence. While you are healthy, make certain key decisions about what sort of end-of-life care you prefer. Otherwise, you will be putting this burden onto your spouse, children, or partner. Additionally, without clear-cut instructions from you, laws in some states make it complicated to withhold or withdraw care even when there is little or no probability of significant functional improvement. Also discuss your personal thoughts and wishes with your family. Generally, you should prepare a set of documents that include advance directives—written instructions on the type and extent of care you wish to receive during grave illness. You should designate a health care proxy, someone who understands and can represent your wishes in the event that you can no longer make those decisions or communicate them. You can also sign a living will, but in most states, the designation of health care agent and alternate is most important, provided that you discuss your wishes with the agent and trust that she or he will honor your wishes. Review your thoughts from time to time, especially if your views or attitudes change. Your doctor must know how to reach your health care agent in an urgent situation.

Establishing a Productive Doctor-Patient Relationship

Doctor-patient interactions have suffered in this era of ever-increasing time pressures. Today's medical encounters are too often characterized by physician dominance and patient passivity, with little opportunity for patients to articulate concerns not specifically related to a question asked. Recently, investigators focusing on physician-patient communication have advocated that physicians develop a style that fosters co-participation and relationship building, in which patients are encouraged to take a much more active role. Arguments abound that the managed care environment, such as HMOs, makes this collaborative approach unattainable, especially for the older patient. However, there is mounting evidence that co-participation and relationship building provide better patient outcomes and greater physician and patient satisfaction and that they actually take no more time than the traditional, rapid-fire question-and-answer approach. The challenge, then, is to adapt the co-participation approach in the context of a circumscribed time frame.

Meeting this challenge is especially important at the initial office visit. We are indebted to Richard Frankel, Ph.D., who has suggested an important strategy to ensure a successful outcome for both the patient and the doctor at the first visit. He advocates a structured approach to the initial office contact with an older person, one that allows the time during the visit to focus on developing a sense of co-participation and relationship building. In our experience, following his approach yields key information essential to making judgments, such as the need for imaging or laboratory testing. The key is for the doctor to take maximum advantage of a patient's summary of information form, which is submitted before the visit. This enables the physician to use the many nonverbal, observational methods of evaluating older patients during the visit itself. This approach is accomplished in the following sequence:

1. Previsit information gathering.
2. Functional status evaluation by observation.
3. Preparation of the environment.
4. Open-ended interview.
5. Limited physical examination.
6. Agreement.

1. Previsit Information Gathering

An organized review of the medical history is necessary before the physician can determine what type of further assessment might be indicated. This is the part of the initial interview that has the potential for consuming the most time. Many elements of the "standard" medical history are easily collected on a structured questionnaire completed by the patient and/or family members before the visit. Health care offices frequently use a standardized form that asks about present medical conditions, significant past illnesses, hospitalizations, surgeries, and allergies, which they often mail or fax to you in advance. You should always complete this document as fully as possible well before the scheduled visit; if you need assistance with remaining parts of it, you may ask the office nurse or assistant while you are in the waiting room.

The content of this "previsit history" will vary from one practice to another, but in a generalist's practice it should be adapted to the older patient. For example, a social history contains information that can relate to an older person's safety. In particular, the physician needs to be able to create a mental image of the living arrangements for each patient. Does she or he live alone? Does she or he require caregiver assistance? Is the patient a caregiver for someone else, such as a grandchild or spouse? Has the patient spent any time in the past year in a nursing home? It is also important to ascertain what role the patient's family members (or others) play in providing health care, managing financial affairs, and/or helping with daily activities of living. Are all these consistent with the patient's desires and preferences and with what the patient tells the doctor during the visit?

Whatever other data elements are selected, a current medication list, including over-the-counter medications, should always be included. A staffperson should encourage the patient to bring all of his or her medications to the initial visit, a technique sometimes referred to as the "shopping bag test." These medications and their uses can be listed before the physician visit. This single practice may be the most cost-effective and potentially beneficial aspect of the history gathering.

The identification of known risk factors for certain diseases (such as a stroke or heart attack) or events (such as a fall or auto accident) has become an issue of increasing importance to health care providers and health insurers alike. When a potential risk factor (for example, frailty) is identified at the time of initial involvement, an assessment process can be initiated and appropriate services offered. Much risk measurement information can be gathered through screening questionnaires that are completed before the initial visit. The previsit history can identify areas where further questioning or assessment is warranted that a busy practitioner might not raise and that the patient might forget to volunteer during the first visit.

2. Functional Status Evaluation by Observation

Much of the "functional status" evaluation is obtained by simple observation of the patient and family in the process of moving from the waiting room to the private office and to and from the examining table. For example, the observant physician can learn a great deal by watching a patient get out of a chair, walk a short distance, and get up onto an exam table. With older patients, the physician or other health care provider watches these movements.

3. Preparation of the Environment

Careful attention must be paid to patients' age-related visual and hearing impairments, which may otherwise contribute to wasted time in the interview setting. Lighting should be bright but without glare, spaces wide and uncluttered, and signage clear and easily read. Background noise from music systems or ventilating fans can interfere with hearing and should be kept to a minimum.

4. Open-ended Interview

The physician's interview technique should be characterized by several qualities: attentive listening, learning the specific reason(s) for the visit, and looking for opportunities to uncover key health-related facts and to express empathy with and compassion for the patient and family.

Physicians dealing with older patients should avoid closed questions (that is, yes/no questions). Because it may take longer for an older person to formulate a thoughtful response, the physician may have a tendency to "move on," so useful information may not be uncovered. Also, physicians sometimes assume that a patient's failure to answer a question promptly is a sign of dementia, when the patient may only be trying to formulate a well-thought-out answer. Misinformation may result from a directive interview style. Even when armed with substantial information obtained before the interview, the physician has to craft the initial encounter. Consider the following closed-end interview:

DOCTOR: It's nice to see you, Mrs. G. Well, it looks like we have a lot of ground to cover. I see you are having problems with your ears?

MRS. G: Something's not right.

DOCTOR: Are you hard of hearing?

MRS. G: What?

DOCTOR: Don't worry; we'll get that checked. Are you ever dizzy?

MRS. G: Sometimes, well, I'm not really sure.

DOCTOR: Does the room spin around, or do you spin?

MRS. G: No, I don't think the room spins.

DOCTOR: Then you feel yourself spinning?

MRS. G: I don't think so. Well, that's not it exactly.

DOCTOR: Well, we have only 20 minutes. We'll get some tests to check that out. Probably nothing serious. You know, lots of people your age have these little problems. Why don't we get going with the rest of this list right from the top?

Now, let's see how an open-ended interview might go:

DOCTOR: Hello, Mrs. G. We have about 20 minutes to get acquainted today, and of course we'll see each other again, but I want to make sure we have time for the things that are important to you. I see from the papers you filled out that you are mainly concerned about your ears.

MRS. G: That's right.

DOCTOR: Uh-huh.

MRS. G: I'm not sure how to describe it.

DOCTOR: Uh-huh.

MRS. G: I can hear OK, but sometimes it sounds like I have a buzzer in my head.

DOCTOR: What do you think is going on?

MRS. G: Oh, you're the doctor.

DOCTOR: (Silence.)

MRS. G: Well, it probably sounds silly, but it happens every time I get a flare of arthritis—probably all in my imagination—just getting old.

DOCTOR: I'm sorry about that. Anything else?

MRS. G: I've tried everything. I take aspirin for the arthritis, and when the noise starts I try taking lots more, but it doesn't help, just seems to get worse.

DOCTOR: It sounds like this has you worried.

MRS. G: Well, so many of my friends are dying of cancer.

The two interview sequences take about the same amount of time but reveal different information. Studies have demonstrated that attentive listening is usually a more efficient method of eliciting information than the rapid-fire question-and-answer approach. Furthermore, if these important issues do not surface early in the visit, they may be "saved up" and expressed just when the physician feels the interview is over. The patient thus feels that he or she has not been listened to, and the physician is left with a sense of frustration.

LEARNING THE REASON(S) FOR THE VISIT

Perhaps the most basic and important information to be obtained is the patient's reason for coming to the office. Is it to establish a medical record and rapport with the new doctor? Is it to obtain referrals to specialists? Does the patient have an acute problem or need to manage a chronic disease? In fact, patients may well have multiple agenda items, and this plurality of needs may not become apparent until the end of the session. Early in the interview, the doctor should ask how the patient perceives his or her health status and what he or she believes is "wrong." Few patients (and *very* few older patients) will spontaneously volunteer their reasons; they tend to wait to be asked. We are learning from contemporary studies, such as the Macarthur Field Studies of Successful Aging, that community-dwelling older persons give very reliable assessments of their own health and health care needs.

SEEKING OPPORTUNITIES TO BE COMPASSIONATE

Studies demonstrate that experienced clinicians are skillful at employing brief "windows of opportunity" to interrupt the flow of the traditional medical interview and focus on the patient's nonmedical agenda. They briefly pursue whatever issues, usually of a psychological or social nature, are important to the patient. These instances offer the physician an opportunity to express empathy with the patient, gain a great deal of initial insight into the patient's problems, and generate substantial satisfaction and trust. Moreover, these interactions can be successfully used even in interviews lasting only 10 to 12 minutes. No encounter is too short to allow the demonstration of kindness and concern. The time available is of less importance than the skills of the clinician. As a patient, if you find a physician lacks these qualities on more than one occasion, you should reconsider working with him or her.

5. Limited Physical Examination

A "complete" physical examination is an oxymoron in any context. What is appropriate is a thoughtfully focused examination prompted by information obtained during the interview portion of the visit. However limited, there should always be some physical examination, including measuring blood pressure and listening to the heartbeat and the lungs, at every visit. These procedures may uncover significant abnormalities and are also reassuring to older patients.

6. Agreement

The interview should never conclude without a plan of subsequent action that is understood and agreed to by the patient and/ or family or caregivers. An example of this might be, "We have agreed to increase your blood pressure medicine to two tablets every morning; you will not add any salt to your food at the table; and I will phone you in two to three days to review your laboratory results from the blood taken today."

In summary, the educated patient will look for all of these characteristics and skills in a health care provider.

11

Screening Tests for Seniors

Certain screening tests are appropriate for older adults. However, considerable judgment is required to make specific suggestions for each patient. These choices of what studies or examinations to order are likely to vary from one patient to another, reflecting the heterogeneity of the older population. Fundamentally, recommendations for each individual need to be based on (a) the person's unique accumulation of illnesses, (b) estimates of the person's level of physiological loss, (c) prediction of the person's life expectancy, and (d) the person's functional limitations, if any.

What does the geriatrician want to know about a new patient? At many medical schools, it is popular to take medical students to a prominent art museum, where a docent is paired with a physician and students are asked to interpret great art, usually portraits. The ostensible purpose of such outings is to extend the powers of observation of these fledgling physicians in a rarefied environment away from the often-stressful atmosphere of their science classes. However, most students believe that the excursion is yet another test of their medical prowess and potential. So when interpreting a copy of the Mona Lisa, for example, one student may point out precancerous blemishes on the face, another might see possible subtle eye problems, and yet another might speculate on the significance of the bleak landscape in the background. Interestingly, when a geriatrician is the teacher on these art museum excursions, he or she typically asks a different set of questions than would another instructor: Does Mona Lisa appear oriented to her surroundings? Is the emotionless smile a sign of depression, or even an attempt to suppress an increasing urge to urinate? What does her grooming tell us about her ability to carry out the ordinary tasks of daily living? Does the virtual lack of eyebrows suggest thyroid deficiency, a common problem in older women? Are there any obstacles in the background that might lead to an injurious fall? This example demonstrates how the health care professionals who care for and advise seniors have a different way of seeing situations and health issues.

Geriatricians and all generalists "see" the human body as substantively more than the sum of its parts and are primarily interested in knowing how well a patient is performing the common activities of daily living. Not surprisingly, therefore, the preventive examination, especially as age advances, becomes more and more concentrated on the mind, muscle function, bones, sight, and hearing. All, of course, are areas critical to the preservation of function and independence. At the same time, there is recognition that some of the most life-threatening disease states, such as some forms of cancer, are far more frequent after age 65, and that modern medicine now has the tools to detect cancer at earlier stages, when it is more amenable to therapy.

Chronological age should not be a de facto barrier to screening or preventive services. However, the primary care provider must apply judgment as to what is or is not recommended for preventive strategies based on each patient's unique circumstance. The clinical course of much chronic illness, such as heart failure, high blood pressure, and diabetes, is somewhat different in the oldest old and requires a different set of diagnostic skills to detect and possibly reverse some of the damage.

The Medicare program has begun to recognize the benefit of a preventive approach, starting with the recent authorization of the "Welcome to Medicare" examination, in which, for the first time, physicians are reimbursed for an evaluation of patients simply because they have reached the age of 65 years. This "Welcome to Medicare" office visit is intended to help health care providers develop a specific plan of screening, immunization, and counseling for their patients. Physicians obtain a medical and social history with special attention to what are described as "modifiable risk factors." Most patients will have a simple screening for depression and an assessment of their functional ability and safety. These observational maneuvers are followed by a targeted physical examination. Patients are then guided to educational resources and, when needed, counseling and referral services. Finally, patients are provided with a written checklist for obtaining preventive services that are covered under Medicare. In addition to screening, this visit is the perfect time to check immunization status for bacterial pneumonia and the influenza and shingles viruses. Medicare will cover this exam if you get it within the first 12 months after enrolling in Part B. You pay 20 percent of the Medicare-approved charge for this exam.

Most authorities suggest annual monitoring of height and weight (for calculation of body mass index, or BMI), blood pressure screening, and referral to an eye professional to test for visual acuity, macular degeneration, and glaucoma. Questionnaires to detect depression and alcoholism are typically administered at varying intervals throughout the course of life, depending on age, gender, and overall health status. Some experts suggest the following: a one-time abdominal ultrasound for males who have ever smoked (to detect weakening and bulging of the abdominal aorta); bone density measurements, especially for women; mammography for women who have an estimated life expectancy of at least 10 years; a Pap smear for women; and screening for colon cancer by direct imaging with colonoscopy. The indications for these tests require considerable individualization and should be discussed with your primary care provider.

Later in the life cycle, preventive attention is redirected increasingly toward functional assessment of both cognitive and physical performance. Simple screening tests of cognition, strength, balance, and flexibility can be performed quickly, accurately, and painlessly in the primary care office setting, as can tests for problems of bladder control.

We are often asked at what age certain screening tests should be eliminated. There are no strict age standards, and the generalist must decide using the criteria stated above. Chronological age should never be the sole determinant of the value of preventive testing or suggested health maintenance strategies. The wise patient therefore should expect such judgment from a health care provider and always some suggestion to at least preserve, if not increase, function. One should not expect the primary care provider to say something is or is not indicated on the basis of age alone. The reality is far more complicated than that.

12

Managing Medications

Patients and their doctors have had something of a love-hate relationship when it comes to medications. One of the most enduring quotes about medication use is attributed to Oliver Wendell Holmes, Sr., a Harvard-trained physician, author, and poet of the nineteenth century: "If the whole materia medica [medical material], as now used, could be sunk to the bottom of the sea, it would be so much the better for mankind—and all the worse for the fishes."

During the past 40 years of our medical careers, we have witnessed the rapid development and deployment of pharmacologic agents that are highly effective in managing chronic diseases, especially cardiovascular disease, osteoporosis, and gastrointestinal distress. Yet, as seasoned geriatricians, we have time after time seen patients cross that thin line between effective drug use and dangerous drug use. More recently, we have appreciated the complexity of getting a simple prescription filled and the often crushing costs of prescription medications, even if patients use the Medicare Part D prescription benefit.

This chapter presents an approach to the use of prescription drugs to assist you in making sound and effective choices. We do not make recommendations for specific drugs; for that advice, you should consult your primary care provider.

Establish Open Communication with Your Health Care Providers

The most important principle to remember is that the safe and effective use of powerful prescription drugs requires an interactive partnership between you (the user) and the health care team. There are many potential barriers to this communication. Time—or, more precisely, lack of time—is perhaps the biggest barrier. For good reasons, electronic prescribing is replacing the handwritten prescription, but as a consequence, there is often little or no face-to-face discussion between the patient and the health provider concerning prescribed drugs. In most large pharmacies, medications are dispensed by a clerk in an atmosphere of rote compliance with federal regulations. The Health Insurance Portability and Accountability Act of 1996 (HIPAA) requires pharmacies to offer consumers the option of discussing the medication in semiprivacy with the pharmacist. However, if the line at the checkout counter is long and everyone in the pharmacy is obviously busy, it may be intimidating or impractical to exercise your right to face-to-face consultation. Of course, if you pick up the medication at the drive-through window, communication options are nil. As an alternative to direct communication, one can always refer to the printed instructions provided with every prescription. But these descriptions are typically very complicated, exhaustive, in small type, and stapled to the bag or envelope in a way that makes it difficult to remove them without tearing. Read without interpretation, they can be frightening. It is essential, therefore, to have a personal and effective approach to managing drug therapy. This requires that we all become better-informed consumers.

Understand How Drugs Work in Your Body

The place to start is with a basic understanding of what happens when our bodies come into contact with a drug, usually through oral intake but also through our skin, through inhalation, or by an injection. Once a drug is absorbed into the body, it is transported to the target organs, where the therapeutic effect takes place. However, it is a rare drug that will not also affect other organs or body processes. For example, an allergy medicine may alleviate a stuffy nose but can also result in bouts of confusion in an older adult. The body degrades the drug and excretes it by breaking it down into smaller molecules, principally in the liver and the kidney. As we age, there is a great deal of variability in kidney and liver function, and this affects drug metabolism. The end result of these changes of aging is that the human body has less tolerance for drug effects. When this reduced tolerance is coupled with the fact that we are often taking multiple drugs that may interact with each other, it is easy to see why older adults are less tolerant of drugs in general. Especially important in this regard is the much higher likelihood of unintentional effects on the functioning of one's brain and nervous system. Thus, when physicians evaluate a patent who complains of confusion or memory problems, they are likely to start with a careful history of all medications the patient is taking. In fact, drug interactions and side effects are so common that almost any time an older person has a new complaint, we assume a drug-related problem until proven otherwise.

Maintain a Personal Medication Record

All drugs have the potential to cause unintended side effects, usually termed "adverse drug reactions." Often these are well beyond the more familiar and transient heartburn or allergies such as rash. Because many of us seniors are taking multiple drugs (six is the average), the chances of complex interactions are more likely. For anyone taking eight or more different prescription drugs daily, there is an 80 percent probability of an adverse drug reaction. It is often not a matter of if, but when, such a reaction will be observed. To best manage personal drug therapy, we therefore need to implement key measures of self-responsibility and communication.

First and foremost, it is essential that we have knowledge about our prescribed drugs, including the name and purpose of the medication, the dosing interval, potential interactions with other drugs or foods, and the reported adverse drug reactions for that agent. You can obtain this information from your physician or designated office staff. Pharmacists can also supply this information. If these routes are not practical, there are many highly reliable sources of information available at no or little cost. The National Institutes of Health maintain an excellent website as part of the Medline Plus information source (www.medlineplus .gov).

Once this information is in hand, you should establish and maintain a personal record of your prescription medications, doses, and time intervals. Any changes can be easily noted. A small notebook is useful for this purpose and should include allergies and the identity and dosages of any over-the-counter medications, vitamins and minerals, and herbal or nonherbal supplements you may be taking. There are also preprinted booklets available for this purpose. A convenient personal medication record form is available from the AARP website (www.aarp.org) and can be filled out electronically or by hand. This record is extremely important, and you should bring it to any appointment with your doctor. Alternatively, consumer-friendly electronic medical records are being developed by Google and Microsoft as well as other companies. If your physician's office is already using electronic medical records, a listing of your medications can be copied for your use, but at present nothing substitutes for a personal record that you take responsibility for keeping up to date. Also, if you are using your primary care physician's record, be certain that it includes any additional medications prescribed by other health care professionals and lists all the over-the-counter medications and supplements that you take frequently.

Managing the Costs of Prescription Drugs

Some people have the misconception that the Medicare prescription benefit (Medicare Part D) covers the total cost of prescription drugs. This is not the case. Under the federal mandates for Medicare Part D, there is a stated obligation for recipients to share in the cost of prescription drugs. The formula is far from simple, and the following explanation is only an approximation. Representative costs are calculated using 2010 cost estimates. Monthly premiums are between $9 and $140 depending on geographical location. There are three components of the coverage plan: an initial coverage limit, catastrophic coverage, and an intermediate gap in coverage (popularly termed the "doughnut hole"). Initial coverage begins with an annual $310 deductible that you pay out of pocket. After the deductible is met, beneficiaries pay 25 percent of covered costs up to the first limit, $2,520 (the sum of what the patient paid and what the plan covered, not including the deductible). After that, the beneficiary pays 100 percent of costs up to the upper limit, $4,550. For you, this means a potential total out-of-pocket payment of over $2,800 per year. At that point, catastrophic coverage activates and the beneficiary pays only 5 percent of subsequent costs for the fiscal year. With the current high cost of drugs, it is relatively easy to reach the "gap." Also, you must factor in the cost of any "nonformulary" (noncovered) drugs you take, as you must pay for them out of pocket. Because brand-name drugs are expensive, it is always an incentive to your health care professional to prescribe generic drugs whenever possible. As of July 2009, the Obama administration has proposed an agreement with major pharmaceutical companies to provide a subsidy to reduce consumer spending in the doughnut hole, which, if it becomes law, may substantially reduce the financial burden for Medicare recipients.

Obtaining Medicare Part D coverage is voluntary and requires enrollment in a designated private plan. Plans can be either stand-alone or part of a Medicare Advantage Plan, which usually bundles medical care costs and prescription drug benefits in a single package. Both of these options may require the patient to pay a premium. Plans vary widely in drug coverage, premiums, and benefits. Many are run by large drugstore chains. Choosing a plan can be a formidable task, but Medicare provides valuable assistance (www.Medicare.gov).

Despite the complexities of drug use and the requisite financial planning, Medicare prescription drug coverage can be a major help for Medicare recipients. However, the partnership between the patient, her or his primary care physician, and the pharmacist is still the most crucial factor in maximizing the benefits of modern drug use.

Of course, pharmaceutical drugs do not work if you don't take them. It is easy to forget a medication from time to time or confuse one medication with another. A number of simple yet effective tactics can minimize this risk. It is common for seniors to be taking multiple medications. As each new drug is added, there is often little consideration of how this agent might complicate the pattern you have already established for taking your medications, especially if you are taking drugs several times daily. If you are in this situation, ask your physician or pharmacist if it might be possible to take a form of drug that can be taken just once a day. If not, perhaps the frequencies of use can be modified so that you will have to remember to take them only two or at most three times daily. Finally, buy one or more of the convenient drug storage boxes so that you can place all of the day's or week's drugs in labeled compartments at one time and then empty the compartments at the labeled time or day. A variety of these containers are available at all pharmacies.

The Influence of the Pharmaceutical Industry

These days, a chapter on taking medications would not be complete without some discussion of the influence of the pharmaceutical industry on you and your doctor. The remainder of this chapter, therefore, explains some potential pitfalls to avoid. At first you may be inclined to skip this section. What could pharmaceutical manufacturers possibly have to do with you and the relationship you have with your physician? The influence of drug marketing is overwhelming, and you are wise to want to understand something about it.

The influence of the pharmaceutical industry on medical practice and potentially on the relationship you have with your physician has increased markedly in recent years. This influence could be good or bad for your personal health care. Knowing something about it will help you obtain the best care from your doctor.

There are many ways this influence plays out on a daily basis; some are subtle and others are obvious.

The reason for the recent increase in the pharmaceutical industry's influence in clinical practice is the federal government's authorization under the Freedom of Information Act of direct-to-consumer advertising of drugs (and other medical therapies). This program has grown substantially in recent years. In an article in the *New England Journal of Medicine* (August 16, 2007), Dr. Julie Donohue and colleagues state that direct-to-consumer advertising expenditures increased from $985 million in 1996 to $4.237 billion in 2005. As large as these figures are, they still represent only 1.3 and 2.6 percent, respectively, of all pharmaceutical industry advertising (the bulk of which is aimed directly at prescribers). So you and all health care providers are inundated with drug company advertisements.

The theoretical benefit of direct-to-consumer advertising is that a consumer can be more informed about illnesses and drugs and this knowledge can lead to intelligent discussions with health care providers. On the surface, this seems sensible and, indeed, does work this way. But in clinical practice there are many problems with this direct appeal to patients. Most direct-to-consumer advertisements are for new drugs, often those that are more expensive than the older drugs. Rarely is there advertising for old, established drugs, which are no longer protected by patent yet still have an important place in therapy. An example of this is the absence in advertising of a stand-alone and no-longer-patented antihypertension drug, hydrochlorothiazide. Yet this agent is one of the mainstay drugs in most hypertension therapy regimens, and current studies continue to confirm its efficacy and value. Indeed, most textbooks and recent scientific review papers recommend it, or a drug similar to it, as the starting point in the treatment of a patient with newly diagnosed hypertension. In advertisements aimed directly at consumers, however, hydrochlorothiazide is not featured. Rather, the advertisement touts the latest addition to a new class of drugs. Notably, new drugs by definition lack the safety records of established generic drugs. The advertisement may also be pushing a new combination (and usually a more expensive formulation) of old drugs. We almost never prescribe combination drugs (two or more drugs formulated into one tablet or capsule). They typically cost more, and when a problem occurs, for example, a side effect, it is difficult to identify which drug caused the problem. In other words, the convenience of a single tablet as opposed to two does not outweigh the cost and risk. For these reasons, we never start two or more drugs simultaneously unless absolutely necessary.

There is clear evidence that direct-to-consumer advertising of drugs is an effective marking strategy. Studies have shown that nearly one-third of individuals who see a drug advertisement for a condition they have will ask their physician about it, and, of those who ask for the drug, almost one in four is given a prescription for it. Indeed, this confirms what we all know: advertising works.

Where direct-to-consumer advertising often has a negative effect is in the clinical encounter between the patient and the health care provider. Time is a precious element in the visit, especially for seniors, who typically have multiple conditions and are taking multiple drugs. It takes considerable time for a physician to discuss with a patient why a newer, prominently advertised drug is not indicated for them or is not the first choice according to published scholarly reviews. If we had ample time, educating patients about the pros and cons of new medications would be a good thing. However, the science underlying these drug differences requires that the patient have a sophisticated understanding of how medications affect their physiological condition. The message of staying with the tried-and-true medication often cannot compete effectively with the flashy advertisements.

Recently, there has been a barrage of advertising for a group of drugs called cholinesterase inhibitors for use in patients with dementia. These drugs theoretically could improve brain function that has been diminished by Alzheimer disease or related dementias by increasing the concentration of chemicals involved in intracellular communication in the brain. Reviewing the advertisements in this area would lead one to believe that the current agents can halt or slow the progress of these diseases and even prevent or delay nursing home placement. When the data are analyzed carefully, they do show a minor and statistically significant improvement on the scores of standard memory-assessment tests. However, the clinical significance of these changes simply is not apparent to most clinicians or family members. Most scholars believe that the published reports that these drugs can delay placement in a nursing home of a person who has cognitive impairment are so flawed that they cannot be trusted. In addition, the drugs are expensive and have significant side effects.

For a physician to discuss these factors and the research related to treating Alzheimer disease fully with a patient and family takes fifteen to twenty minutes or longer. When time during an office visit is limited, it often is easier to write the prescription. Giving a prescription based on a drug company's advertisement may then lead to its long-term use even as the disease is progressing. Most geriatricians believe that a trial of three or four months of a cholinesterase-inhibiting drug for the treatment of a patient with Alzheimer disease occasionally may be appropriate, but there must be a clear plan to discontinue it if no benefits accrue or if side effects are witnessed. Even this strategy requires clear communication between the health care provider and the patient and family. Unfortunately, we have seen patients admitted to a nursing home who had advanced dementia and continued to take a cholinesterase-inhibiting agent that had been prescribed years earlier and continued even in the presence of deteriorating mental function. This situation creates a potential side effect burden and considerable expense with no benefit.

While direct-to-consumer advertising of drugs can alert the public to the availability of new drugs and provide information about a disease, its primary purpose, understandably, is to sell drugs. Such advertising does sell drugs, but in general the pharmaceutical industry and its shareholders benefit more than patients. So the wise consumer will be cautious about drug advertisements. When talking to any doctor, the consumer should have a reasoned discussion about the drug and avoid health care providers who simply write a prescription (or, worse, give out samples) with no meaningful explanation.

13

Nutrition and Exercise

When Dan Buettner, author of the book *Blue Zones,* began his exploration of key communities around the world reputed to enjoy remarkable longevity and quality of life during aging, he found key distinguishing aspects of lifestyle which were common to these groups. Despite differing genetic heritage and despite living on different continents, these populations seemed invariably to eat a diet relatively lower in calories than diets in most of the developed world. They also got more exercise. These real-world observations correlate very well with a large body of scientific information suggesting that control of body weight and maintenance of activity not only reduces the severity of cardiovascular disease but also lengthens life. Therefore, following proven principles of nutrition and physical activity tops the list of effective measures anyone can adopt. If we explore some of the changes in body composition that frequently occur as we age, you will appreciate that nutrition and activity are interrelated. Most important, these changes are not inevitable and can be ameliorated in most cases by applying knowledge of sound nutrition and physical activity. Increasing scientific evidence strongly suggests that, even if you have never paid much attention to body weight or have been a "couch potato," adopting sound principles can have profound benefits, even in your 60s, 70s, 80s, and beyond.

When we think of nutritional issues contributing to poor health in seniors, the usual image is that of a malnourished older person. While such nutritional deficiencies can be serious, especially in extreme old age, by far the more common and dangerous nutritional problem for seniors in the United States is being overweight or even obese. Studies of the "obesity epidemic" have concentrated on younger people and paid less attention to understanding the frequency and clinical consequences of excess weight in those age 65 or older. In fact, 25 percent of adults between the ages of 60 and 69 years are obese, as are 17 percent of those older than 70. These statistics have implications far beyond a person's appearance. Excessive body weight contributes to stress injury of major joints, like knees, which ultimately will limit physical activity. Excessive body fat contributes to inability of the body to produce enough insulin, and diabetes is a frequent consequence. Also, obesity often leads to a rise in blood pressure, and hypertension is the consequence. Abdominal fat is associated with higher levels of inflammation, contributing to damage to blood vessels, cardiovascular disease, and possibly cancer and cognitive disorders.

Let's review some of the common changes in the composition of our bodies as we age. At about age 40, we usually begin a process of losing muscle and gaining fat throughout the body. The loss of muscle accelerates in the 60s and 70s in both men and women. Because we tend to build up a surplus of muscle in youth, initially we are unaware that muscle strength is lessening. For a while, body weight may not change. At the same time, there is a loss of bone tissue—more pronounced in women after menopause—which can lead to osteoporosis, which men as well as women can develop. During the initial stages, these various changes are not evident. Because muscle has a much higher metabolic rate than fat tissue, once these changes take place, our caloric needs are reduced, and if we continue to consume the same amount of calories, we accumulate additional fat.

There are often many barriers to achieving sound nutrition. Healthy eating can be expensive, especially for those living alone. Fortunately, there are many sources of dietary information aimed at the needs of older adults. For example, the U.S. Department of Agriculture provides an excellent and authoritative starting point for understanding food groups and meal portions as part of the My Pyramid program available electronically (www.mypyramid .gov) or in print. In general, the components of a sound diet are somewhat age specific and include, for older adults, attention to the basic six food types essential to a healthy diet (grains and fiber, vegetables, fruits, dairy products, protein from beans and lean meat, and liquid vegetable oils). The My Pyramid program allows personalized calculation of a typical diet based on age, body weight, and caloric needs. Of course, any modification of your usual diet should be done only with the knowledge and supervision of your physician.

We want to interject a cautionary note regarding the use of various fad diets and unconventional nutritional supplements. Ask your doctor before spending money on such products. They may be worthless, have subtle but unpleasant side effects, or even be dangerous.

One of the most important advances in our understanding of the aging process is that we now know the value of continued physical activity. We mentioned above that muscle mass decreases with age. Let's explore this phenomenon in greater depth. Studies of "average people" have shown that, beginning around age 30, about 0.5 percent of muscle mass is lost per year through age 50. Then, in those who remain relatively inactive, another 30 percent is lost from age 50 to 70. Cardiovascular capacity to respond to physical demands, sometimes called aerobic capacity, drops as well, as does the ability to maintain good balance.

Here is the important point. For many years it was assumed that these considerable changes were an inevitable part of the aging process. It turns out that this isn't so. Scientific work over the past 20 years has unequivocally demonstrated that these dramatic declines in muscle and strength are mostly due to decreased physical activity. These age-related changes can be significantly reduced by a prudent program of physical activity (in addition to that required for basic activities of daily life). This exceptionally good news has only slowly permeated into clinical practice, and some physicians are still reluctant to advise programs of physical exercise for seniors.

Talk with your physician about a sensible exercise program tailored to you. It is important to consider any barriers to exercise that may apply in your case. In the majority of cases, there will be no barriers, and an increase in physical activity will pay off enormously. A sound exercise routine should include activities that develop strength, endurance, and flexibility and that restore muscle mass. Most important, a program is most likely to succeed if it is enjoyable. Make it fun.

The general recommendations for exercise suggest 30 minutes of at least "moderately intensive" exercise at least 5 days a week. However, good results have been observed with a minimum of 20 minutes of walking three days a week, plus 20 minutes of weights, balance, and flexibility twice weekly. Some exercise is better than none, and in all cases the activity should include some form of exercise against resistance or with weights. A good guide to exercise is published by the National Institute on Aging (*Exercise: A Guide from the National Institute on Aging*, NIH Publication 02-4258). The entire guide can be found at www.nia.nih.gov. Print copies are available for a small charge.

Scientists have also demonstrated that simple changes in daily habits can increase your physical activity and benefit your health substantially. Try these simple strategies: use the stairs instead of the elevator or escalator, park farther away in the parking lot, walk all the aisles when food shopping, and walk whenever the distance is less than five blocks, as long as the area is safe.

If you are not active now, be sure to discuss any exercise plans with a health care professional. You should expect to encounter some hindrances to beginning and sustaining a program of physical activity. Some commercial gyms cater to a young population, and many seniors feel uncomfortable in this type of environment. Talk to friends about establishments that have programs and facilities targeted to older adults. Many hospitals and nonprofit organizations, such as the YMCA or community centers, have excellent programs. Another common barrier is a negative body image. However, a trip to any modern sports store will allow anyone to pick out suitable exercise "gear" that will allow movement while hiding those parts of the anatomy that may cause excessive self-awareness. Of course, an excellent program can be done at home, and some people prefer privacy, but part of the fun of exercise is getting out with others, listening to music, and moving about! Also, many people find that a commitment to exercise with others motivates them on days when they might otherwise skip exercising.

Almost all older adults who take up an exercise program consisting of brisk walking, simple weight training, and flexibility exercises for 6–8 weeks describe a sense of renewed energy and mental alertness that serves as a lasting incentive. Beyond that, weight control will be easier, and often diabetes can be better controlled, even enough to permit a reduction in medication. Similarly, people with high blood pressure will often experience some normalization of blood pressure. Many people report better sleep. Over the long term, the medical benefits of physical activity include better heart health, lower risk of stroke, less pain from arthritis, and possibly some improvement in memory and thought processes.

Now get moving and take charge of your health!

Index

AARP, 8, 39, 58, 105
activities of daily living, 129
ADGAP (Association of Directors of Geriatric Academic Programs), 101–2
advance directives, 119–20
ageism, 116–17
age-related diseases, 10
aging: perceptions of, 3–9; successful, 10–13
aides, personal, 43
alcoholism, 130
Alzheimer disease, 4, 6, 44, 141
American Association for Long-Term Care Insurance (AALTCI), 31
American Association of Homes and Services for the Aging, 39
American Association of Medical Colleges, 104
American Geriatrics Society (AGS), 105
anemia, 7, 15
aorta, abdominal, 131
arthritis, 5, 18, 148
artworks, observation of, 128–29
assisted living, 37, 40, 43

assisted living facilities, 23, 35–36, 40
athletes, 16
Atlantic Philanthropies, 100, 103, 104

baby boomers, 100, 109
balance, 131, 146
Baltimore Longitudinal Study of Aging (BLSA), 15
bladder control, 3–4, 9, 131
blood pressure: and exercise, 148; high, 130; and hypertension, 18, 30, 77, 139, 144; increases in, 9; medication for, 139–40; and obesity, 144; and physical examination, 130; record of, 112
blood sugar level, 19
blood vessels, 144
body mass index (BMI), 112, 130
body weight, 13; control of, 143, 144; and exercise, 148; gain or loss of, 9, 33; management of, 112–13; monitoring of, 130; and nursing homes, 33
bone density, 131, 145

bone fracture, 15
brain disease, 6
breathing. *See* respiratory capacity
Buettner, Dan, 12, 143
Bureau of Health Professions, 69

California, 12
cancer, 4, 7, 8, 9, 44, 129, 131, 144
cardiac recovery, 42
cardiology, 70, 100
cardiovascular disease, 143, 144
cardiovascular function, 5, 146
care, 14–19; community-based, 41;
    coordination of, 45, 53, 61; pre-
    ventive, 36, 51; quality of, 18;
    transitions of, 46–48. *See also* phy-
    sicians, primary care; primary care
care managers/case managers, 45–46
care plan: and hospice, 44; individ-
    ual, 14, 18; transfer-related prob-
    lems with, 47
catheter, bladder, 33
Centers for Medicare and Medicaid
    Services (CMS), 32, 46, 104
chest pain, 17
children, 17, 60
cholinesterase inhibitors, 141–42
chronic diseases, 8, 9, 24, 53, 54, 57
clergy, 44
cognition. *See* mental function/
    cognition
colonoscopy, 131
colostomy, 42
computed tomography (CT) scans,
    63, 78, 80
concerns, list of, 117–18
concierge medicine, 73
consultants, 72, 91, 92, 97
continuing care retirement
    communities (CCRCs), 24, 35, 37–
    39, 40
co-participation, 120–21
coronary artery disease, 5, 61
Costa Rica, 13
costs: to business, 51; diagnostic, 49;
    of drugs, 132, 136–38; health care,

49–50; and hospitals, 51–52;
    insurance, 31–32; Medicare, 51,
    52; physician, 71; therapy, 49
creativity, 6–7
cross-sectional studies, 7, 15

day care centers, 23, 24, 25, 40–41
delirium, 102. *See also* mental
    function/cognition
dementia, 19, 30, 141
Dennis W. Jahnigen Career Develop-
    ment Scholars Award Program,
    102–3
dentists, 64
Department of Agriculture, 145
Department of Veterans Affairs, 32,
    35, 36, 47, 104
depression, 77, 130
dermatology, 103
diabetes, 18, 19, 42, 77, 112, 130,
    144, 148
diagnosis, 75–79; by generalist vs.
    specialist, 87–88; and health care
    costs, 49; individual, 18
diagnostic caution, 78
diagnostic tests and procedures, 66,
    121; complications from, 9, 62,
    63, 77–78; different responses to,
    17; and hospice care, 45; imaging
    in, 55, 63, 77, 78, 79–80, 121;
    injury from, 88; and Medicare, 53,
    55; and physical reserve, 16;
    records of, 112; results of, 79–80,
    92, 93; and screening tests, 128–
    31; and specialists, 92, 93–94
diet/nutrition, 13, 19, 62, 143–44,
    145
disability/disabilities, 57, 74;
    disease-related, 11; multiple
    chronic, 24; and rehabilitation
    centers, 29–30; and successful
    aging, 11
diseases, 8; age-related, 10; chronic,
    8, 9, 24, 53, 54, 57; and longevity,
    12; low risk of, 11; pandemic,
    17–18; and successful aging, 11;

understanding of, 110–11. *See also* illnesses; illnesses, chronic

diversity/heterogeneity, 14, 18–19, 77

Donald W. Reynolds Foundation, 100

drug plan providers, 55–56

drugs/medication: advertising of, 139–42; attention to taking of, 137–38; careful monitoring of, 27; change in, during hospitalization, 27; communication about, 133, 140–42; consultant advice about, 92; cost of, 132, 136–38; erection-enhancing, 6; and exercise, 148; generic, 137; interaction of, 135; management of, 132–42; and Medicare, 53, 55–56; nonprescription, 111, 119; in office visit discussion, 122; personal record of, 112, 122, 135–36; and physical reserve, 15; processing of prescriptions for, 66; regular review of, 62; risks of, 17, 102; safety of, 140; and shopping bag test, 111, 122; side effects of, 119, 135, 140; tolerance for, 134; understanding of, 111, 118–19, 134, 135; for urinary incontinence, 4. *See also* pharmaceutical industry; *specific drugs*

education: and home care, 42; multidisciplinary, 103; about urinary incontinence, 4. *See also* medical schools

emergency departments, 51, 52, 62

emergency response systems, 48

emergency rooms, 65

endocrinology, 100

end-of-life issues, 119–20

enteral therapy, 41

environment, 12

equipment, home medical, 42

erectile dysfunction, 6

exercise, 62; benefits of, 5, 112, 113, 146–48; and diabetes, 19; and longevity, 13, 143–44

eyesight. *See* vision/eyesight

family: and diagnosis, 77; discussion of end-of-life issues with, 119; initiation of specialist consultation by, 96–97; and patient social history, 122; and team care, 64; and transfer-related problems, 47–48

family physicians, 40, 60, 66

fee-for-service healthcare, 67–68, 73

flexibility, physical, 131

Foundation for Health in Aging, American Geriatrics Society, 105

Frankel, Richard, 120–21

functional ability: assessment of, 118; and home care, 42; lessening of, 9–10, 29; limitations in, 118, 128; observation of, 123; and preventive examinations, 129, 130, 131; review of, 62. *See also* physical function

gastroenterology, 100

general internists, 60

genetics, 12

Geriatric Education Center (GEC) program, 69

geriatricians, 8, 36, 60; as consultants, 72; as generalist primary care providers, 72; income of, 70; shortage of, 70, 71–72, 74, 99–105

geriatrics: competency of physicians in, 74; education in, 99–105; and multidisciplinary team education, 69; and patient-generated requests for consultation, 97; research in, 104; as specialty, 71; team care in, 64; and thoughtfulness of consultant, 91; training in, 72–73

glaucoma, 130

glucose control, 18–19

government, 43, 57–58, 67

graduate nursing assistants (GNAs), 34
grief counselors, 44
guided care, 68–69
gynecology, 103

health: assessment of, 61; multiple problems with, 17–18, 61, 88, 91; responsibility for, 109–13. *See also* diseases; illnesses; illnesses, chronic
health care: and care managers, 45–46; cost of, 49–50; and costs to business, 51; education of physicians about, 23; financing of, 49
health care organizations, 67
health care plans, 55
health care providers: contact information for, 112; and exercise, 5; and urinary incontinence, 4
health care proxies, 120
health care reform, 51, 57–59, 116
health maintenance, 61
health maintenance organizations (HMOs), 55, 115–16, 120
health records, 111–12. *See also* medical records
Health Resources and Services Administration (HRSA), 69, 101
hearing, 9, 18, 118
heart, enlarged, 7, 15
heart attack, 17
heart disease, 44
heart failure, 61, 130; congestive, 30
height, 130
hemoglobin A1C, 18–19, 112
heterogeneity/diversity, 14, 18–19, 77
high blood pressure. *See* blood pressure
home: evaluation of situation in, 81–82; hospice care in, 43, 44; remaining in own, 40. *See also* living arrangements
home health aides, 41
home health care, 41–43; and hospice care, 44; and Medicare, 55; nonskilled, 41, 43; skilled, 41

home medical equipment, 42
hormone injections, 6
hospice care, 43–45, 55
hospital groups, 58
hospitalists, 26–27, 29, 95–96
hospitals, 24, 25–29, 36; capacity of, 51–52; charity, 53; and continuing care retirement communities, 37; discharge summary from, 30; as financial component of health care, 25; and health care costs, 51–52; and hospice care, 43; interns and resident doctors at, 28; and Medicare, 53, 54, 55; and nursing homes, 34; selection of, 54; teaching, 27–29; and team care, 64; and transfer of information, 27; and transfer-related problems, 27, 48. *See also* medical centers
house calls, 80–83
hydrochlorothiazide, 139–40
hypoglycemia, 19

illnesses: acute, 42, 54, 55; and aging, 8; atypical presentation of, 17; catastrophic, 53; complications from, 9; and emergency departments, 52; and home care, 42; multiple, 17–19, 29–30, 53, 62, 77, 80; and rehabilitation centers, 29–30; responses to, 14; and screening tests, 128; terminal, 43; understanding of, 110–11. *See also* diseases
illnesses, chronic: and aging, 14, 17–19; and emergency department, 52; and hospice, 44; and Medicare, 42; in oldest old, 130; and poverty, 53; and Program of All-Inclusive Care for the Elderly, 36; and visits to physicians, 80. *See also* diseases
immunization, 62, 130
independence, 37, 39, 42, 129
information, transfer of, 27, 47–48
infusion treatments, 41, 42
Institute of Medicine, 101

insulin, 19, 144

insurance: and assisted living facilities, 36; capitated or prepaid, 68; and care managers, 45; cost of, 31–32; and health care costs, 51; and home care, 42; and hospice and palliative care, 43; lack of, 51; life care, 39–40; long-term care, 31–32, 36, 37, 43; and medical day care, 40; Medigap, 54, 56; and nursing home care, 31

insurance companies, 58

interns, 28

intestinal bleeding, 7

Italy, 12

Japan, 12

John A. Hartford Foundation, 100, 103, 104

Kahn, Robert L., 11, 12

kidneys, 16, 17, 19

life expectancy: changes in, 67, 100, 109; and exceptional longevity, 11–13; and hospice care, 43–44; and lifestyle, 143; and Medicaid, 57; and Medicare, 53, 54, 57; and screening tests, 128, 131

lifestyle, 143

Lindenauer, Peter, 26

living arrangements, 122. *See also* home

living wills, 120

longevity, 11-13. *See also* life expectancy

longitudinal studies, 7, 15

long-term care, 31–32, 36, 37, 43; and community-based care, 41; and Medicare, 53; and Medicare A, 55

lung disease, 44, 77. *See also* respiratory capacity

Macarthur Field Studies of Successful Aging, 126

macular degeneration, 130

mammography, 131

managed care, 68, 97, 114, 120

media, 4, 10, 139

Medicaid, 57, 74; and community-based care, 41; and medical day care, 40; and nursing home care, 31; and poverty, 54; and Program of All-Inclusive Care for the Elderly, 36

medical centers, 25–29, 35, 41. *See also* hospitals

medical clinics, 34

medical day care facilities, 40–41

medical device manufacturers, 58

medical history, 121–22, 130

Medical Homes, 46, 68–69, 110

medical records, 47, 94, 111–12

medical schools, 28, 99–105; faculty at, 70

medical students, 28–29, 70–71

Medicare, 67, 73, 74; and care management, 46; and health care costs, 51, 52; and home care, 41, 42, 44; and hospice care, 43, 45; key components of, 54; and medical day care, 40; and medication, 136–37; and nursing home care, 31; open enrollment period for, 56; and palliative care, 43; Part A, 54–55; Part B, 55, 56, 130; Part C, 55; Part D, 55–56, 132, 136–37; and physician costs, 71; and preventive health benefit, 56–57, 130; and Program of All-Inclusive Care for the Elderly, 36; reimbursement rates for, 58; strengths and weaknesses of, 52–57; and transfer-related problems, 47; types of coverage under, 54–55

Medicare Administration, 56

Medicare Advantage Plan, 55, 68, 137

Medicare Rights Center, 56

medication. *See* drugs/medication

memory, 141, 148; and aging, 3; difficulties with, 9; and disease, 6; and medication, 134
meningitis, 53
menopause, 145
mental function/cognition, 6, 131; disorders of, 144; and exercise, 5, 148; impairment of, 3, 10, 18; limitations in, 118; and medication, 134, 141; and normal aging, 15; stimulation of, 112, 113; and successful aging, 11. *See also* delirium; dementia; memory
mental health care, 55
multidisciplinary care, 68–69
multidisciplinary medical practice, 78
muscle mass, 144–46
muscle strength, 5, 131, 144, 146
My Pyramid program, 145

National Adult Day Services Association, 41
National Institute on Aging (NIA), 8, 15, 69, 147
National Institutes of Health (NIH), 15, 69, 103, 104, 111, 135
nerve conduction time, 7, 16
neurodegenerative disease, 6
neurosurgery, 103
nurse practitioners, 24–25, 26, 27, 60; solo, 66, 67; and team care, 64, 65, 73
nurses, 28; and assisted living facilities, 35; as care managers, 45; and continuing care retirement communities, 37; and home health care, 41, 42; hospice, 44, 45; nursing home, 33, 34; nursing home care training for, 34–35; as partners with physicians, 68; and rehabilitation centers, 29; and team care, 64–65, 73
nursing facilities, 55
nursing homes, 23, 24, 30–35, 36, 74; challenges of care at, 34; custodial service in, 31–32; evaluation of, 32–35; and exercise, 5; and hospice care, 43; inspection of, 32, 33; kinds of, 31; and life care insurance, 40; and medical centers, 25; and medical day care, 40; and Medicare Part A, 55; and Medicare Part B, 55; payment for care at, 31–32; questions for visits to, 33–34; skilled service, 31; and social history, 122; staff salaries at, 34; staff-to-resident ratios at, 32; staff turnover rate at, 34; and subacute rehabilitation programs, 30; transfer from hospitals to, 27; and transfer-related problems, 48

obesity, 13, 112–13, 144
obstetricians, 100
occupational therapy, 29, 41
office visits, 117–20, 122, 136
ophthalmology, 100, 103
orthopedic surgery, 100, 103
osteopathic schools, 71
osteoporosis, 145
ostomy care, 42

palliative care, 43–45
Pap smears, 131
Parkinson disease, 11
patient summary of information form, 121
Paul B. Beeson Career Development Award Program, 104
pediatrics, 17, 60, 100
personality changes, 4–5
pharmaceutical industry, 58, 138–42. *See also* drugs/medication
pharmacists, 42, 56, 64, 68, 111, 135
physical examinations, 127, 130
physical function, 11, 118, 131. *See also* functional ability
physical therapy, 29, 41, 45, 103
physician assistants, 25, 26, 27, 60, 64, 65, 73
physicians: attending, 28; consulting, 29; family, 40, 60, 66; and health

care reform, 58; and home health care, 41, 42; and hospitalization, 26–29; and malpractice lawsuits, 78; and Medicare, 54, 55; and Medicare Part B, 55; nursing home care training for, 34–35; and partnership with nurses, 68; and Program of All-Inclusive Care for the Elderly, 37; and rehabilitation centers, 29; selection of, 54; solo, 66, 67; and team care, 64, 65

physicians, generalist, 26, 60–61, 63, 70; costs of, 71; income of, 70, 71; percentage of seniors as patients of, 100; perspective of, 75–85; role of and relationship with specialists, 91–92, 93; shortage of, 74

physicians, primary care, 60; and acute illness, 67; and care management, 46; choice of, 114–15; communication with, 116–17, 118, 120; compassion of, 126–27; and continuing care retirement communities, 39; decreasing numbers of, 51, 67; diagnosis by, 75–79; examination by, 127; follow-up visits with, 79–80, 88–89; and home care, 42–43; and hospice care, 44, 45; and hospital care, 27, 28; hospitalists, 26–27, 29, 95–96; house calls by, 80–83; knowledge of, 24; learning from patients by, 83–85; listening by, 124–26; and Medicare preventive health benefit, 57, 130; office environments of, 123; office visits with, 117–20, 136; open-ended interviews with, 123, 124–26; openness with, 119; perspective of, 75–85; and pharmaceutical industry, 138; qualifications of, 110, 115; reasons for visits with, 126; recommendations about, 114–15; relationship with, 61–63, 67, 75–76, 84–85, 110, 115–17, 120–27; retirement of, 110, 114; role of and relationship

with specialists, 86–89, 90, 93–97; shortage of, 25, 69–73; solo, 66; structure of initial visit with, 121–23; and team care, 73; and transfer-related problems, 47, 48; and transfer to rehabilitation centers, 30

physicians, specialist, 73, 86–98; accessibility and punctuality of, 90–91; co-management with, 95–96; communication with, 88, 89–90, 93–96; and diagnostic procedures, 63, 92, 93–94; focus of, 91–92; and generalist physicians, 60, 61, 63, 66; humility of, 92–93; ideal consultations with, 89–93; income of, 70; patient/family initiated consultations with, 96–97; patient perception of, 92–93; percentage of seniors as patients of, 100; practicality of, 92; and primary care physicians, 24; questions for, 87; role of, 86–89; as teachers, 97–98; thoughtfulness of, 91

physiological function: and aging, 8; changes in, 8, 10, 14, 15–17, 19; decrease in, 7–8, 9–10, 62, 77, 128

physiological reserve, 14, 15–16, 61, 63

pneumonia, 130

politicians, 58

polymyalgia rheumatica, 77

poverty, 53, 54, 57, 74

preexisting health conditions, 56

preferred provider organizations (PPOs), 55

prescriptions, 66

preventive services/care, 51, 57, 62, 129–30, 131; and Medicare, 54, 55

primary care, 60–73; access to, 62; crisis in availability of, 69–73; and geriatrics, 72; and health care reform, 58; as keystone of health care system, 24; low prestige of,

primary care *(cont.)*
72; as national goal, 73; number of trainees in, 70; office-based, 26; patient-centered, 67; team care in, 64–69. *See also* physicians, primary care
privacy, protection of, 47
Program of All-Inclusive Care for the Elderly (PACE), 36–37, 40, 68–69, 74
psychologists, 64

quality of care, 18

radiology, 103
red blood cell count, 7, 15
rehabilitation centers, 29–30; acute, 29; subacute, 29–30; transfer from hospitals to, 27; and transfer-related problems, 48
rehabilitation services, 55
religious lay persons, 44
residency training, 28
residential facilities, 64
residents, 28; covering, 28
respiratory capacity, 7, 16. *See also* lung disease
respiratory care, 41
respiratory disease, 18
retirement communities, 38. *See also* continuing care retirement communities
rheumatoid arthritis, 11
risk factors, 122–23, 130
Rowe, John W., 11, 12

screening tests, 128-31
senility, 15
sensory disease, 6
sexuality, 5–6
shingles virus, 130
side effects, 119, 135, 140
skin wrinkles, 9
smoking, 131; avoidance of, 13
social history, 122, 130

Social Security, 55
social workers, 25, 29, 33, 41, 44, 45
speech therapy, 29, 41
states/state government, 41, 58, 71
stroke, 4
studies, cross-sectional and longitudinal, 7, 15
successful aging, 10–13
sugar, 112
supplements, 111
surgeons, 86
surgery, 9, 15, 28, 100, 102, 103
symptoms and signs, atypical presentation of, 17. *See also* diagnosis; *specific problems*

team care, 64–69
T. Franklin Williams Scholars Program, 104
therapeutic procedures: complications from, 62; risks from, 78
therapy, 68; and health care costs, 49; and home health care, 41, 42; individual, 18; occupational, 29, 41; physical, 29, 41, 45, 103; and team care, 64
thoracic surgery, 103
thyroid problems, 4
transfer-related problems, 27, 47–48
transportation, 13, 36, 41, 43

urinary incontinence, 3–4, 9
urology, 100, 103

vaccination, 33, 130
veterans, 32
Veterans Affairs (VA) Medical Centers, 101
vision/eyesight, 7, 9, 16, 18, 118, 130
vitamin B12 deficiency, 4
vitamins, 4, 111, 119

wills, living, 120
women, 3, 103, 145
wound care, 42

About the Authors

JOHN R. BURTON

My career started with medical school at McGill University, followed by training in internal medicine at the Baltimore City Hospitals. These years of training were interrupted by two years in the Air Force, serving at the Clark Air Force Base Hospital in the Philippines. During the Vietnam conflict I was asked to assist the only nephrologist in the hospital because of the large number of soldiers who had developed acute kidney failure from trauma or illness. I became profoundly interested in nephrology, so when I left the military and finished two years of residency at the Baltimore City Hospitals, a career in nephrology dominated my planning. Accordingly, I did a year of specialty training in nephrology at Massachusetts General Hospital. In 1972, I joined the faculty of Johns Hopkins University in nephrology, working primarily at the Baltimore City Hospitals.

My role as a consultant in nephrology was to provide specialty advice to patients and their physicians about kidney and/or fluid and electrolyte problems. Invariably patients came to me with a specific issue or question carefully refined by previous physicians or other health care professionals. A typical initial comment from a patient was, "My doctor is concerned about my potassium (or kidney function or urinalysis or blood pressure or sodium concentration or infections) and wanted advice." The statement was never "I'm tired" or "I feel weak" or something similar. I became fascinated with what medicine would be like in the role of the first person to hear a patient's concern and then try to figure out what was wrong and serve as the patient's medical advisor and advocate over time. I missed close physician/patient bonds and personal relationships that, while possible as a consultant, were uncommon even when seeing a patient frequently over time.

I longed to experience medicine through the lens of primary care. When I presented these thoughts to my department chair, he thought they were interesting and could lead to a needed community and medical center resource. So in 1974, I entered a recently established community-based health care office. It was instantly the most exciting, challenging, and professionally rewarding experience in my career.

At first, the practice consisted of typical internal medicine, except that many patients were older. Without any training in geriatrics, I was building a practice of mostly older individuals who lived in the community. As the practice grew, other faculty physicians were attracted to the group and physicians-in-training began to request clerkships with us.

In time, my colleagues and I recognized that many patients arrived by wheelchair or even stretcher, often with two or three family members along to help them. Accordingly, we decided that it would be better for these essentially homebound patients and their families if we saw them at home. Thus, in the 1970s, we launched a physician house call program. As that grew, it became an attractive site for physicians-in-training and for medical student teaching. After several years in our community site, my colleagues and I were invited to move the practice to the medical center campus and were encouraged to further develop the Division of Geriatric Medicine, started in the 1950s by the late Dr. Mason F. Lord. I was able to qualify by experience to become certified in geriatric medicine by the American Board of Internal Medicine soon after such examinations were offered.

WILLIAM J. HALL

I am a born-again geriatrician. My incubation period covered half of my professional career before I realized that caring for older adults was my true calling.

I had no exposure to grandparents or other older persons during my early youth. While in medical school at the University of Michigan in the 1960s, there was no such thing as a geriatrics rotation, and few faculty members were interested in the care of elderly patients.

I moved to New Haven, Connecticut, for my residency in internal medicine and, as was common at that time, my training was interrupted for military service. I found myself assigned to the U.S. Public Health Service and stationed in Hiroshima, Japan. There, along with Japanese physicians, I participated in the biennial clinical evaluation of a large cohort of individuals enrolled in the famous study evaluating the biological effects of human exposure to ionizing radiation—the survivors of the atomic bombs dropped on Japan. This was my first "practice." Most of the participants were older, and, because my Japanese language skills were not very well developed, I was forced to rely on clinical observation more than conventional history taking. In retrospect, this experience was the beginning of my geriatrics training.

I returned to New Haven to complete my residency at Yale and subsequently moved to the University of Rochester School of Medicine, where I trained in pulmonary disease and remained on the faculty, caring for mostly older patients in the clinic and intensive care units. Eventually, I became chief of medicine at a large community hospital in Rochester. In that capacity, I was challenged by long acute hospital stays of older patients and the three D's: delirium, depression, and dementia. I helped establish a social day care program for frail elderly people, and before I knew it, I was a full-time geriatrician.